EMOTIONAL HYGIENE

The No-Nonsense Guide to Love, Boundaries, and Self-Respect

By T Light

Published by The Crackajack Company

Table of Contents

Introduction: Why Emotional Hygiene Matters

You brush your teeth every day, right? You shower (hopefully). You wash your hands before eating. Nobody throws you a parade for these things because they're just... what you do. Basic human maintenance. We call it hygiene, not because it's glamorous, but because it's essential.

Now here's the fun part: emotional hygiene works exactly the same way. Except most of us never learned it. We got a million lectures about flossing, but zero about how to spot when someone's slowly draining your life force like an emotional vampire. (And yes, those are real. You probably know three.)

Here's what nobody tells you: most people's emotional hygiene is... let's just say not the standards you are entitled to or deserve. We let anyone into our inner circle like it's an open-door policy at a supermarket. We recycle the same arguments with different people. We mistake intensity for intimacy, chaos for chemistry, and someone's neediness for love. We're out here confusing guilt with obligation like they're the same thing. (Spoiler: they're not.)

This guide isn't about fixing you, because,and you better believe this, you are not broken. You're just operating with some outdated software that got installed a long time ago. Somewhere along the way, you picked up some very creative ideas about what love means, what you owe people, and what you're allowed to want for yourself. This book? It's the software update.

Emotional hygiene is about prevention, not damage control. It's about spotting the red flags before you're six months deep in a situationship with someone who 'doesn't do labels' but somehow has very strong opinions about who you can follow on Instagram or what you wear to the dinner party. It's about knowing when to exit stage left, when to speak up, and when to stop explaining yourself to people who've already decided you're the villain in their story.

Let's get something straight: this isn't about becoming one of those cold, walled-off people who treat human connection like a potential liability. Good boundaries don't make you less loving. They just mean you're not handing out unlimited access passes to people who haven't earned them. Self-respect doesn't make you selfish. It makes you honest. And honestly? That's refreshing.

If you're reading this, something brought you here. Maybe you're exhausted from relationships that take way more than they give. Maybe you keep meeting the same person in different bodies. Maybe you're tired of being the only one who seems to care about... well, anything. Maybe you looked around one day and thought, 'How did I end up here again?'

Welcome. That awareness? That little voice saying 'something's not right here'? That's your emotional immune system waking up. Now let's teach it some kung fu.

PART ONE:
THE FOUNDATIONS

Chapter 1: Understanding Emotional Hygiene

Think of emotional hygiene as your daily check-in system. Like running diagnostics on your phone, but for your soul. It's about regularly asking yourself, 'Hey, how are we doing in here?' and actually listening to the answer instead of drowning it out with Netflix, social media, or that third glass of wine.

The goal? Catch the small stuff before it becomes big stuff. You wouldn't wait until your teeth fall out to start brushing, right? Same principle here. Don't wait for a full emotional crisis, a panic attack in the grocery store, or a complete breakdown at your desk to start paying attention to your needs.

Emotional hygiene means noticing when you're playing mental gymnastics to explain away someone's sketchy behaviour. It means catching yourself mid-excuse when you're about to do something that makes you feel icky inside. It means recognizing when you're running on empty, and actually doing something about it instead of just drinking more coffee and hoping for the best.

What Emotional Hygiene Actually Is

Emotional hygiene is the practice of regularly checking in with yourself, identifying what's yours to carry and what isn't, and taking action before small problems become chronic conditions.

It's about asking yourself questions like: 'Why do I feel anxious every time this person texts me?' Or 'Why do I dread Sunday dinners with my family?' Or 'Why do I feel guilty for taking a break when I've been working nonstop for weeks?' And then, here's the revolutionary part, actually answering those questions honestly instead of brushing them off with 'it's fine' or 'that's just how things are.'

Most people treat their emotional health like they treat that weird noise their car makes. Ignore it and hope it goes away. Spoiler alert: it doesn't. It just gets louder until something breaks down completely. Then you're stuck on the side of the emotional highway wondering how you got here.

Emotional hygiene is proactive maintenance. It's checking the oil before the engine seizes. It's noticing the warning signs before the breakdown. It's boring, unglamorous, daily work that prevents dramatic disasters.

But here's the thing about preventive maintenance: nobody notices when it works. Nobody congratulates you for the crisis that didn't happen. Nobody sees the relationships you didn't ruin because you caught yourself before you snapped. Nobody applauds the boundaries you held that prevented resentment from building.

That's okay. You're not doing this for applause. You're doing it because you're tired of cleaning up preventable messes.

The Five Pillars of Emotional Hygiene

Emotional hygiene rests on five foundational practices. Master these and everything else becomes easier.

1. Awareness: Knowing what you're actually feeling

Most people have no idea how they actually feel most of the time. They've been performing emotions for so long that they've lost touch with the real ones underneath.

You say you're 'fine' when you're exhausted. You say you're 'tired' when you're actually depressed. You say you're 'stressed' when you're furious. You've learned to translate your actual emotions into more socially acceptable versions.

Awareness means cutting through that translation layer. It means sitting with yourself long enough to figure out what you're actually experiencing, not just what you think you're supposed to be feeling.

This is harder than it sounds. Your mind will resist. It will offer you comfortable lies. 'I'm just tired.' 'I'm being too sensitive.' 'It's not that bad.' Don't let it. Push past the automatic responses and get to the truth underneath.

Here's how to practice awareness: Set a timer for two minutes. Sit somewhere quiet. Close your eyes. Ask yourself: 'What am I actually feeling right now?' Don't judge it. Don't fix it. Just name it. Anxious. Angry. Sad. Overwhelmed. Numb. Whatever it is, name it.

Do this daily. Eventually, you'll get faster at it. Eventually, you won't need the timer. Eventually, you'll be able to check in with yourself in real-time, mid-conversation, mid-conflict, mid-crisis.

That's when awareness becomes a superpower.

2. Boundaries: Protecting your energy and wellbeing

Boundaries are not walls. They're not about shutting people out or being cold or unavailable. Boundaries are simply information: here's what works for me, here's what doesn't, here's where I end and you begin. Here is the line I'm comfortable with. Step beyond this and I have to push you away for my own peace.

Most people think boundaries are mean. They're not. Boundaries are kind. To yourself and to others. They let people know how to be in relationship with you. They prevent resentment from building. They create the container for healthy connection.

Good boundaries look like: 'I'm not available after 9 PM.' 'I don't lend money.' 'I need advance notice for plans.' 'That topic isn't up for discussion.' 'I'm leaving if you continue to speak to me that way.'

Notice these aren't requests. They're statements. You're not asking permission. You're providing information about your limits.

Boundaries feel uncomfortable at first. Especially if you've spent your whole life having none. You'll feel selfish. Mean. Difficult. Push through it. That discomfort is just old programming telling you that your needs don't matter. Your needs matter.

Start small. Pick one boundary. Maybe it's not responding to texts after a certain time. Maybe it's saying no to plans you don't want to attend. Maybe it's ending conversations that make you uncomfortable. Start there. Get comfortable holding that one boundary. Then add another.

3. Self-honesty: Telling yourself the truth about what's happening

Self-honesty is brutal. It means admitting when you're staying in a situation that's harming you. It means acknowledging when you're making excuses for someone's bad behaviour. It means recognizing when you're the problem.

Most people lie to themselves constantly. 'It's not that bad.' 'They're going through a lot.' 'It'll get better.' 'I'm probably overreacting.' These lies protect you from having to make hard choices, but they also keep you stuck.

Self-honesty means dropping the pretence and facing reality. Yes, it's uncomfortable. Yes, it means you can't keep avoiding what needs to change. That's the point.

Here's the test: if you wouldn't tolerate this behaviour from anyone else, why are you tolerating it from this person? If your best friend came to you with this exact situation, what would you tell them? If you're making excuses for someone's treatment of you that you'd never accept from a stranger, you're lying to yourself.

Self-honesty requires courage. It requires being willing to see what you've been avoiding. It requires admitting uncomfortable truths: that relationship isn't healthy, that job is draining you, that friend only calls when they need something, that pattern keeps repeating because you keep allowing it.

But here's what happens when you get honest with yourself: you stop wasting energy on denial. You stop making excuses. You stop pretending things are okay when they're not. And that clarity? That clarity creates space for actual change.

4. Action: Actually doing something with your awareness

This is where most people get stuck. They have awareness. They know their boundaries. They can see the truth. But they don't act on it.

Action means: leaving the relationship that's draining you, enforcing the boundary someone keeps testing, having the hard conversation you've been avoiding, stopping the pattern you keep repeating, asking for what you need, saying no when you mean no.

Action is where change actually happens. Everything before this is just information gathering. Action is the implementation.

And yes, action is scary. Action has consequences. Action means people might be upset. Action means things might change. Good. Things need to change. That's why you're here.

Start with small actions. You don't have to blow up your entire life in one day. Maybe your action is responding 'I'll think about it' instead of automatically saying yes. Maybe it's leaving the family dinner an hour early. Maybe it's telling someone 'That doesn't work for me' instead of going along with their plan.

Small actions build confidence. Small actions show you that boundaries don't kill you. Small actions prove that you can survive disappointing people. Small actions add up to big changes.

5. Consistency: Doing this daily, not just when you're in crisis

Emotional hygiene is a practice, not an event. It's something you do every single day, even when things are going well. Especially when things are going well.

Most people only pay attention to their emotional health when they're in crisis. When the relationship implodes. When the anxiety becomes unbearable. When they can't get out of bed. But by then, you're in damage control mode. You're cleaning up a mess that could have been prevented.

Consistency means daily check-ins. Weekly assessments. Monthly reviews. Constant recalibration. It's boring. It's repetitive. It works.

Think of it like physical fitness. You don't go to the gym once a year and expect to be healthy. You go regularly. Consistently. Even when you don't feel like it. Especially when you don't feel like it.

Same with emotional hygiene. You check in daily. You maintain your boundaries consistently. You practice self-honesty even when it's uncomfortable. You take small actions regularly instead of waiting for a crisis to force big ones.

Consistency is what transforms knowledge into results. Consistency is what makes emotional hygiene a lifestyle instead of just a concept you read about once.

What Emotional Hygiene Is NOT

Let's clear up some misconceptions right now, because the internet has gotten very creative with what 'self-care' and 'boundaries' supposedly mean.

It's not about being selfish. Taking care of yourself doesn't mean you stop caring about other people. It means you stop setting yourself on fire to keep everyone else warm. There's a difference.

Selfish means you prioritize yourself at the expense of others. Self-care means you prioritize yourself so you can show up for others without resenting them. One destroys relationships. The other sustains them.

You can care deeply about people and still have boundaries. You can love your family and still limit contact. You can be a good friend and still say no sometimes. These things are not mutually exclusive.

It's not about avoiding all discomfort. Growth is uncomfortable. Change is uncomfortable. Healthy conflict is uncomfortable. Emotional hygiene doesn't mean you run from every hard conversation or difficult feeling. It means you learn to tell the difference between productive discomfort and destructive discomfort.

Productive discomfort is growth. It's setting a boundary with someone you love. It's having the conversation you've been avoiding. It's sitting with anxiety instead of numbing it. This discomfort has a purpose. It's moving you toward something better.

Destructive discomfort is harm. It's tolerating abuse. It's staying in situations that actively damage you. It's sacrificing your wellbeing for someone else's comfort. This discomfort serves no one. It's just suffering for the sake of suffering.

Emotional hygiene teaches you to embrace productive discomfort while ending destructive discomfort. That distinction matters.

It's not about perfection. You're going to slip. You're going to cave on a boundary. You're going to people-please when you swore you wouldn't. That's called being human. Emotional hygiene is about catching yourself sooner, recovering faster, and learning from the pattern instead of beating yourself up about it.

Perfectionism is just another form of self-betrayal. It sets impossible standards and then punishes you for being human. Emotional hygiene is about progress, not perfection.

You will mess up. Often. The goal isn't to never mess up. The goal is to mess up less frequently, catch yourself faster, and learn from it instead of repeating the same pattern indefinitely.

It's not a substitute for therapy. If you have trauma, mental health conditions, or serious emotional struggles, you need professional help. Emotional hygiene is a daily practice that complements therapy, not replaces it. Think of therapy as major surgery and emotional hygiene as taking your vitamins. You need both.

Therapy helps you understand the roots of your patterns. It helps you process trauma. It helps you develop new coping strategies. Emotional hygiene helps you implement those strategies daily. It helps you maintain the progress you make in therapy. They work together.

Don't use emotional hygiene as an excuse to avoid getting professional help if you need it. And don't feel like you've failed if self-help practices aren't enough. Sometimes you need more support. That's not weakness. That's wisdom.

It's not about cutting everyone off. The internet loves to scream 'cut them off!' at the first sign of conflict. But healthy emotional hygiene sometimes means staying and working through things. Sometimes it means renegotiating terms. Sometimes it does mean leaving. The point is you're making an intentional choice based on your wellbeing, not running on autopilot or reacting from fear.

'No contact' is a tool, not a solution. Sometimes it's the right tool. Often, it's not. Emotional hygiene teaches you how to discern the difference.

Sometimes the healthiest thing is to maintain the relationship with better boundaries. Sometimes it's to reduce contact. Sometimes it's to end it entirely. But you're making that choice consciously, not reactively.

Why You Never Learned This

Here the hard fact: most people's parents didn't teach them emotional hygiene because most people's parents didn't know it themselves. They were too busy teaching you to be polite, get good grades, and not embarrass the family in public.

You learned to share your toys, not to protect your peace. You learned to respect authority, not to trust your gut. You learned to keep the peace, not to speak up when something felt wrong. You learned to be a good kid, not to honour your own needs.

And somewhere in all that socialization, you absorbed some very specific lies:

- Your feelings are an inconvenience to other people
- Saying no makes you a bad person
- Other people's comfort matters more than your boundaries
- If you're a good person, you'll tolerate bad behaviour
- Keeping the peace is more important than keeping your sanity
- Love means unlimited access and zero boundaries
- Asking for what you need is selfish
- Your worth depends on how useful you are to others
- Conflict is dangerous and should be avoided at all costs
- You're responsible for everyone else's feelings

These aren't truths. They're programming. And like any bad code, they'll crash your system if you don't debug them.

Your parents taught you what they knew. And what they knew was probably pretty limited when it came to emotional health. They were products of their own upbringing, carrying forward the same dysfunctional patterns that were handed down to them.

This isn't about blaming them. It's about understanding where your programming came from so you can choose to reprogram yourself.

The Cost of Ignoring Emotional Hygiene

What happens when you ignore your emotional health? When you keep pushing through? When you keep tolerating what shouldn't be tolerated?

Eventually, your body keeps the score.

Chronic stress becomes anxiety disorders. Suppressed emotions become depression. Unprocessed trauma becomes PTSD. Constant boundary violations become deep shame and worthlessness. Persistent self-abandonment becomes burnout, resentment, and disconnection from yourself.

Your relationships suffer. You attract people who take advantage because you haven't learned to protect yourself. You push away healthy people because you don't know how to accept genuine care. You repeat the same dysfunctional patterns over and over, wondering why you keep ending up in the same situations with different people.

Your work suffers. You burn out. You can't focus. You make mistakes. You feel resentful about things you agreed to. You quit jobs impulsively or stay in toxic environments way too long because you don't trust yourself to make good decisions.

Your physical health suffers. Chronic stress manifests as physical symptoms. Headaches. Digestive issues. Insomnia. Weakened immune system. Chronic pain. Your body is literally trying to tell you something needs to change, but you keep ignoring it.

The cost is high. Higher than most people realize until they're already paying it. Until they're sitting in a doctor's office wondering why they're sick all the time. Until they're alone wondering why all their relationships failed. Until they're exhausted wondering why they have no energy left for the things they used to love.

Don't wait until the bill comes due. Start paying attention now.

The Promise of This Work

Here's what changes when you commit to emotional hygiene:

You breathe easier. Literally. The constant tension in your chest loosens. You're not carrying everyone else's problems anymore. You're not holding your breath waiting for the next crisis. You're not bracing yourself against the next boundary violation.

Your relationships improve. The good ones get better because you're no longer resentful. You're showing up authentically instead of performing. You're giving from a full cup instead of an empty one. The bad ones either improve or end, and both outcomes are wins.

You sleep better. You're not lying awake replaying conversations, worrying about other people's problems, or anxious about tomorrow's obligations you wish you'd said no to. Your nervous system finally gets to rest.

You have energy. Actual energy. Not the fake energy you get from coffee and anxiety. Real energy that comes from not being emotionally drained constantly. Energy for hobbies. For creativity. For joy. For things that actually matter to you.

You like yourself more. Because you're finally acting in alignment with your values instead of betraying yourself daily to keep the peace. Because you're honouring your word to yourself. Because you're treating yourself like someone who matters.

You attract better people. Because you're no longer tolerating terrible treatment, you create space for people who actually know how to treat you well. You stop being a magnet for takers and start being a magnet for reciprocal, healthy relationships.

You feel alive. Not just surviving. Not just getting through the day. Actually alive. Present. Connected to yourself and to life. Able to feel the full range of human emotion instead of just numbness and occasional panic.

That's what's waiting for you on the other side of this work.

How to Start

Don't try to overhaul your entire life today. That's overwhelming and unsustainable.

Start with awareness. Just start noticing. Notice when you feel anxious, resentful, drained. Notice which people, situations, and obligations consistently make you feel worse. Notice the patterns. Notice when you abandon yourself. Notice when you betray your own needs to accommodate someone else.

That's it. Just notice for now. Don't try to fix anything yet. Just pay attention.

Because you can't change what you can't see. And right now, you're operating on autopilot. Emotional hygiene starts with waking up. With becoming conscious of patterns, you've been unconsciously repeating for years, maybe decades.

Set aside two minutes tomorrow morning. Before you check your phone. Before you start your day. Just two minutes to ask yourself: How do I actually feel? What do I need today? What am I carrying that isn't mine?

Two minutes. That's all. Start there.

The good news? You can unlearn this stuff. It takes work. It takes practice. It takes being willing to disappoint people who've gotten very comfortable with you having no boundaries. But it's possible.

And that's what the rest of this book is about.

Chapter 2: The Daily Practice of Honouring Yourself

Knowledge is great. Understanding is wonderful. But neither matters if you don't actually DO anything with it. This chapter is about turning emotional hygiene from a concept into a practice. Something you do daily, like brushing your teeth, except way more likely to actually improve your life.

Here's the uncomfortable truth: reading about emotional hygiene won't change your life. Just as reading a book on swimming will not save you from drowning in the ocean. Only practicing emotional hygiene will change your life. And practice means daily, consistent action even when you don't feel like it.

The practices in this chapter are simple. Not easy, but simple. You don't need special equipment. You don't need to carve out hours. You just need to be willing to check in with yourself consistently and actually honour what you find.

The Morning Check-In (2 Minutes)

Before you grab your phone. Before you check email. Before you dive into everyone else's needs and demands. Two minutes with yourself. Just two. You can do two.

This is the foundation of everything else. This is where you stop, breathe, and actually ask yourself what's happening in your internal world before you start managing everyone else's external world.

Most people wake up and immediately start consuming. Consuming news, consuming social media, consuming other people's opinions and problems and drama. They fill their head with everyone else's noise before they've even checked in with their own signal.

Don't do that. Start with yourself first.

Question 1: How do I actually feel right now?

Not 'fine' (we're all fine, sure). Not how you think you should feel. Not how you'll feel after coffee. Right now, in this moment, what's happening in your body? Anxious? Annoyed? Excited? Tired? Sad? Hopeless? Weirdly optimistic? Dreading something specific? Name it without judgment.

Your body is always giving you information. Most people just ignore it until it starts screaming. That tension in your shoulders? That knot in your stomach? That vague sense of unease you can't quite name? That's data. Pay attention to it.

Don't overthink this. Your first instinct is usually right. If you immediately thought 'anxious' but then tried to talk yourself into 'I'm just tired,' go with anxious. Your mind will try to protect you from uncomfortable truths. Don't let it.

And here's the key: name the emotion without trying to fix it. Don't jump straight to 'okay, I'm anxious, what can I do about it?' Just name it. Acknowledge it. That's enough for now.

Why does this matter? Because most people are so disconnected from their emotions that they don't realize they're stressed until they're having a panic attack. They don't realize they're angry until they're yelling at someone. They don't realize they're sad until they can't get out of bed.

Daily emotional awareness prevents that. It catches feelings when they're still manageable. It gives you information before the crisis hits.

Question 2: What do I need today to not lose my mind?

Be specific. 'Self-care' is too vague. Do you need a nap? A walk? Twenty minutes of silence? A good laugh? Permission to say no to something? Time to yourself before you have to be 'on' for everyone else? An actual meal instead of coffee and anxiety? Figure it out and, here's the radical part, actually do it.

Most people skip this step because they think their needs are negotiable. They're not. Your needs are as legitimate as everyone else's. You just haven't been treating them that way.

This isn't about being indulgent or treating yourself. This is about survival. This is about figuring out what you need to function like a human being instead of a robot that runs on caffeine and resentment.

And yes, sometimes what you need is impossible to get. You can't take a nap when you have back-to-back meetings. Fine. But at least acknowledge that you need it. At least stop lying to yourself that you're fine when you're running on fumes.

Acknowledging an unmet need is still valuable. It helps you understand why you're feeling the way you're feeling. It helps you plan for when you can meet that need. It stops you from blaming yourself for being human.

Here's what happens when you consistently ask yourself what you need: you start actually meeting those needs. You start protecting your energy. You start saying no to things that drain you. You start prioritizing rest, connection, joy. Whatever it is you've been neglecting.

And over time, you stop running on empty all the time.

Question 3: What am I carrying that belongs to someone else?

Your mom's anxiety about your life choices? Your partner's bad mood? Your friend's crisis that somehow became your emergency? Your boss's unrealistic expectations? Your sister's drama that she keeps dumping on you like you're an emotional landfill? Your coworker's stress that they keep making your problem?

Put it down. Not your circus, not your monkeys. This doesn't make you a bad person. It makes you someone with boundaries.

Here's how to tell if you're carrying someone else's emotional baggage: if you're more worried about their problem than they are, it's not yours. If you're spending more energy trying to fix their issue than they are, it's not yours. If your mood is determined entirely by their mood, you're carrying their stuff.

Putting it down doesn't mean you don't care. It means you care enough about yourself to not take on responsibility for things you can't control.

Most people were trained from childhood to be emotional pack mules. You were taught to manage your parents' moods. To fix your siblings' problems. To absorb your family's stress. And you brought that pattern into adulthood, where you're now managing everyone's emotions except your own.

Stop. Their feelings are their responsibility. Their problems are their responsibility. Their life choices are their responsibility. You can care without carrying. You can support without taking on their burden.

This morning check-in takes literally two minutes. You spend more time choosing an Instagram filter. Your emotional health is worth at least that much, yes?

Why Two Minutes Matters

Two minutes sounds insignificant. It is insignificant. That's the point.

Most people don't do emotional check-ins because they think it needs to be this big, formal meditation practice. Thirty minutes of journaling. An hour of reflection. A whole morning devoted to self-care.

No. Two minutes. That's it.

Because two minutes is doable. Two minutes doesn't require motivation or inspiration or the perfect circumstances. Two minutes just requires that you care enough about yourself to spend 120 seconds checking in.

And here's what happens: those two minutes change your entire day. Because you started with awareness instead of reactivity. Because you acknowledged your needs instead of suppressing them. Because you put down what wasn't yours instead of carrying it all day.

You make better decisions. You set better boundaries. You notice patterns sooner. You catch yourself before you snap at someone. You recognize when you need a break before you burn out.

Two minutes of prevention saves hours of damage control.

The Evening Audit (5 Minutes)

End-of-day check-in time. Think of it like checking your bank balance, but for your energy and boundaries. These aren't rhetorical questions. Actually answer them. Write them down if you need to.

The evening audit serves a different purpose than the morning check-in. The morning is about setting intentions and identifying needs. The evening is about learning from what happened. It's about pattern recognition. It's about understanding why you keep making the same choices even when they don't serve you.

Question 1: What drained me today?

Which conversations left you feeling like someone vacuumed out your soul? Which tasks made you want to fake your own death? Which people left you feeling worse than before you interacted with them? Which obligations made you resentful?

Be specific. Don't just say 'work' or 'my family.' What about work? Which tasks? Which meetings? Which interactions? What about your family? Which conversations? Which dynamics? Which expectations?

If the same names keep showing up on this list, that's not coincidence. That's data. Use it. You don't have to immediately cut people off (despite what the internet says), but you do need to notice the pattern and decide what you're going to do about it.

Some drains are unavoidable. Yes, you have to work. Yes, you have to deal with difficult clients sometimes. Yes, family obligations exist. Fine. But at least be honest about what's draining you so you can plan accordingly.

Other drains are completely optional. That friend who only calls when they need something? The family member who makes every conversation about their problems? The social obligation you agreed to but don't actually want to attend? Those are choices. And you can choose differently.

Here's what to do with this information: limit your exposure to the drains you can control. Set boundaries around the ones you can't eliminate entirely. And for the truly toxic ones, the relationships that consistently take more than they give, start considering whether they need to end.

Question 2: Where did I betray myself today?

Did you laugh at a joke that actually made you uncomfortable? Say yes when your whole body was screaming no? Stay quiet when you wanted to speak up? Agree to plans you have zero interest in? Pretend to be fine when you were decidedly not fine? Make excuses for someone's bad behaviour? Accept less than you deserve? Compromise your values to keep the peace?

It happens. We all do it. Just notice it. You can't change patterns you won't acknowledge. The goal isn't perfection. It's awareness. You're building the muscle of recognizing when you're abandoning yourself in real-time.

And here's what's important: don't judge yourself for it. Don't add guilt on top of self-betrayal. Just notice. 'Huh, I did that thing again. I said yes when I meant no.

Interesting. Why did I do that? What was I afraid would happen if I'd been honest?'

Self-betrayal usually comes from fear. Fear of conflict. Fear of disappointing someone. Fear of being alone. Fear of being seen as difficult. Once you understand the fear driving the betrayal, you can address the fear instead of just continuing the pattern.

Here's an example: You say yes to hosting a family dinner even though you're exhausted and don't want to. Why? Because you're afraid if you say no, they'll think you don't care about the family. You're afraid of being labelled as selfish or difficult. You're afraid of the guilt trip that will follow.

Now that you've identified the fear, you can address it directly. Is that fear rational? Is it true that saying no to one dinner means you don't care? Is it true that having boundaries makes you selfish? Or is that just old programming?

Usually, it's just old programming. And once you see it clearly, it loses some of its power.

Question 3: What gave me life?

What made you feel more like yourself and less like an overworked, under-appreciated robot? What made you laugh? What made you feel connected? What made time disappear in a good way instead of a dissociative way? What energized you? What filled your cup instead of draining it?

More of that, please. Life's too short to not do the things that make you feel alive. And if you can't think of anything that gave you life today, that's important information. It means you're running on fumes and need to make some changes.

This question is crucial because it's so easy to focus only on what's wrong, what's draining, what needs to be fixed. But you also need to notice what's working. What's good. What fills you up. Because you need more of that.

And if there's genuinely nothing on your list most days? That's a five-alarm fire. That's your soul trying to tell you that something fundamental needs to change about how you're living your life.

Pay attention to patterns here too. If the same activities, people, or experiences consistently show up on your 'gave me life' list, that's data. Make time for those things. Protect that time. Prioritize it. Not as a reward for getting everything else done, but as a necessary part of being human.

The Weekly Reset (15 Minutes)

Once a week, ask yourself the questions that require a little more honesty and a lot more courage. Sunday evenings work well for this, but pick whatever day makes sense for you.

The weekly reset is where you zoom out from the daily details and look at the bigger picture. You're not just asking what happened today. You're asking what patterns are emerging over time.

Question 1: Am I doing all the work in my relationships?

Not looking for perfect 50/50 here. Life happens, people have seasons. But if you're consistently giving 80% and getting back 20%, that's not a relationship. That's you volunteering at someone's emotional food bank. For free. Forever.

Are you always the one initiating? The one planning? The one checking in? The one remembering birthdays and important details? The one making an effort? The one compromising? The one apologizing? The one trying to make things work?

If you stopped reaching out, would this relationship even exist? That's the real question. And if the answer is no, you need to seriously consider whether this is a relationship worth maintaining.

These are uncomfortable questions. Ask them anyway. Because one-sided relationships will drain you dry. And you deserve reciprocity.

Here's what to do with this information: Talk to the person. Set clear expectations. 'I've noticed I'm always the one initiating. I need this to be more balanced.' See how they respond. If they step up, great. If they make excuses or get defensive or continue the pattern, that tells you everything you need to know.

Some people will rise to meet you. Others won't. Both responses are valuable information.

Question 2: What patterns keep showing up?

Same fight, different person? Same type of chaos, new name? Feeling overlooked in the same ways? Dating the same unavailable person in a different body? Having the same argument with your mother that you've been having for fifteen years? Attracting friends who take but never give? Ending up in jobs where you're overworked and underappreciated?

Your patterns are trying to tell you something. Maybe it's time to listen instead of just hitting repeat and hoping for a different outcome.

Patterns exist because they served a purpose once. They were survival strategies that made sense in context. The parentified child becomes the adult who can't say no to requests for help. The scapegoated child becomes the adult who accepts poor treatment. The golden child becomes the adult who can't stop performing.

Understanding your patterns doesn't mean you're stuck with them. But you can't change what you can't see. So, look. Really look at the patterns you keep repeating. What are they trying to protect you from? What old wound are they trying to avoid reopening? What are they costing you now?

Once you see the pattern clearly, you can interrupt it. You can choose differently. You can try a new response. You can break the cycle.

But first, you have to see it.

Question 3: Which boundary did I let slide this week?

Where did you give someone access they hadn't earned? Where did you accept behaviour, you said you wouldn't tolerate? Where did you ignore your gut because you didn't want to seem difficult? Where did you cave to pressure? Where did you sacrifice your needs for someone else's comfort?

And, here's the real question, why? Fear of being alone? Fear of conflict? Fear of seeming 'difficult'? (Newsflash: 'difficult' often just means 'has standards.')

Understanding why you cave on your boundaries is more important than beating yourself up for it. You can't fix what you don't understand.

Maybe you let your mother guilt you into visiting when you had other plans. Maybe you let your friend cancel on you last-minute for the third time without saying anything. Maybe you let your boss pile more work on you when you're already overwhelmed. Maybe you let your partner speak to you in ways you'd never tolerate from anyone else.

Notice it. Name it. Understand why it happened. Then decide what you're going to do differently next time.

And here's the key: actually do something different next time. Awareness without action is just interesting information. Action is what creates change.

The Monthly Deep Dive (30 Minutes)

Once a month, do a deeper review. Look at the bigger picture. Assess whether your daily practices are actually working or if you need to adjust.

Questions to consider:

• Are my relationships generally improving or declining?

• Am I honouring my boundaries more consistently or less?

• What behaviours have I successfully changed?

• What patterns am I still stuck in?

• What needs to shift in my life right now?

• Am I moving toward the life I want or away from it?

• What am I tolerating that I shouldn't be?

• What am I avoiding that needs to be addressed?

This isn't about judging yourself. It's about honest assessment. Progress isn't linear. Some months you'll backslide. That's normal. The point is to notice and course-correct, not to achieve perfection.

Use this monthly review to celebrate wins too. Did you hold a boundary you would have caved on before? Did you say no without guilt? Did you have a hard conversation you've been avoiding? Did you end a relationship that wasn't serving you?

Those are victories. Acknowledge them. You're changing lifelong patterns. That deserves recognition.

Making It Stick

Here's the thing about daily practices: they only work if you actually do them. Revolutionary concept, I know.

Start small. Don't try to overhaul your entire emotional life in one day. Pick one practice, maybe just the morning check-in, and do it consistently for a week. Then add the evening audit. Then the weekly reset.

You're building a habit. Habits take time. Research says anywhere from 21 days to 254 days, depending on the complexity. Be patient with yourself. Be consistent. Be willing to feel awkward and uncomfortable at first.

And here's what you'll notice: the more you check in with yourself, the less you'll betray yourself. The more you honour your needs, the less resentful you'll feel. The more you protect your boundaries, the better your relationships will get (or the clearer it will become which ones need to end).

This is how you take your life back. Not through one big dramatic gesture, but through small, daily acts of self-honouring that add up over time.

You'll miss days. You'll skip the practice sometimes. You'll fall back into old patterns. That's fine. That's human. Just start again the next day. Don't use one missed day as an excuse to give up entirely.

The goal isn't perfection. The goal is consistency over time. It's showing up for yourself more often than you abandon yourself. It's choosing yourself a little more each day until choosing yourself becomes automatic.

Start today. Two minutes. You've got this.

Chapter 3: How We Learn to Betray Ourselves

Nobody wakes up one day and decides, 'You know what? I'm going to completely abandon my own needs and make everyone else's comfort my full-time job.' It doesn't happen like that. Self-betrayal is learned. It's taught. And it usually starts in childhood, handed down like a family recipe nobody asked for.

Here's the uncomfortable truth: the people who loved you the most probably also taught you how to betray yourself. Not because they were evil. Not because they didn't care. But because they were operating from their own programming, their own unhealed wounds, their own survival strategies that they mistook for love.

And now here you are, an adult, repeating patterns you didn't even know you learned. Abandoning yourself in ways that feel automatic because you've been doing it so long you forgot there was another way.

This chapter is about understanding where those patterns came from. Not so you can blame your parents or play victim. But so you can see the programming clearly enough to decide whether you want to keep running it.

The Family System That Raised You

Every family has a system. Spoken and unspoken rules about what's acceptable, what gets you praised, what gets you punished, and what never, ever gets talked about. These rules shape you way more than any parenting book or therapy session.

In healthy family systems, children are allowed to have needs, express feelings, make mistakes, and develop their own identities. Their worth isn't conditional on performance, compliance, or emotional management of the adults around them. They're taught that they matter. That their feelings are valid. That they don't exist to serve others.

In unhealthy family systems (which is... most of them, honestly), children learn that love is conditional. That their value depends on being useful, convenient, quiet, successful, or whatever specific flavour of achievement their parents needed to feel okay about themselves.

You learned what made the adults comfortable and what made them uncomfortable. And if you're someone who struggles with boundaries now, you learned early that making adults uncomfortable was dangerous. So you got really, really good at reading the room, managing moods, and making yourself small.

You became an expert in other people's emotions and an amateur in your own. You learned to prioritize their comfort over your authenticity. You learned that your role was to regulate their nervous system, not honour your own.

And that training? That's still running. You're still reading the room. Still managing moods. Still making yourself small. Just now you're doing it with partners, bosses, friends, and strangers instead of parents.

The Lessons That Stuck

Here are some of the most common lessons people learn about self-betrayal in childhood. See which ones feel familiar:

'Your feelings are too much.' Maybe you cried too loudly. Maybe you got excited about the 'wrong' things. Maybe you were told to 'calm down' or 'stop being so sensitive' every time you had a normal human reaction to things. You learned that your emotional responses were a problem that needed to be managed, hidden, or suppressed.

So now, as an adult, you apologize for crying. You downplay your excitement. You minimize your pain. You've internalized the message that your emotions are an inconvenience to others, so you hide them. You perform 'fine' even when you're falling apart inside.

The cost? You're disconnected from your own emotional reality. You don't trust your feelings. You second-guess your reactions. And other people learn that they can treat you poorly because you won't make a fuss about it.

'Love means sacrifice.' You watched your mother give up her dreams for the family. You saw your father work himself to death for people who didn't appreciate it. You were told that 'real' love requires you to put yourself last, always. You learned that wanting things for yourself was selfish.

So now you confuse self-abandonment with love. You think that if you're not suffering for someone, you must not really care about them. You believe that sacrifice is proof of devotion. You give and give and give until you're resentful and empty, and then you wonder why your relationships aren't fulfilling.

The truth? Real love doesn't require you to destroy yourself. Real love is reciprocal, sustainable, and honours everyone's needs. Including yours. What you learned wasn't love. It was co-dependency dressed up in noble language.

'Conflict is dangerous.' Maybe your parents fought constantly and it was terrifying. Maybe they never fought and swept everything under the rug until it exploded. Either way, you learned that expressing needs, setting boundaries, or saying no created conflict. And conflict felt like the end of the world.

So now you avoid conflict at all costs. You agree to things you don't want. You stay quiet when you should speak up. You let people walk all over you because confronting them feels impossible. You'd rather betray yourself than risk an uncomfortable conversation.

The problem? Avoiding conflict doesn't prevent it. It just delays it. And all that unexpressed anger, resentment, and frustration? It's eating you alive from the inside.

'Your worth is conditional.' Love came with strings attached. Praise came with expectations. Attention was something you earned through good grades, good behaviour, or being whatever version of yourself made the adults proud. You learned to perform instead of just be.

So now you're constantly performing. Trying to earn love through achievement. Trying to prove your worth through productivity. Terrified that if you stop being useful, people will stop caring about you. You can't just exist. You have to justify your existence through constant doing.

The exhaustion is real. And so is the fear underneath it: what if I'm not lovable just as I am? What if my worth really is conditional? What if I stop performing and everyone leaves?

'Other people's emotions are your responsibility.' When mom was upset, you had to fix it. When dad was angry, you had to manage it. Your job wasn't to be a kid.

It was to be an emotional support animal for adults who should have been supporting you.

So now you feel responsible for everyone's emotions. If someone's upset, you assume it's your job to fix it. If someone's angry, you assume you caused it. You can't separate their feelings from your responsibility. You absorb their moods like a sponge and spend all your energy trying to regulate them.

The reality? You're not responsible for anyone else's emotions. Not your partner's. Not your parents'. Not your friends'. Not your boss's. Their feelings are theirs to manage. Your job is to manage your own.

The Parentified Child

Parentification is when children are forced to take on adult emotional or practical responsibilities way before they're developmentally ready. It's one of the fastest ways to teach someone to abandon themselves.

Maybe you were the mediator between fighting parents. Maybe you took care of younger siblings while your parents checked out. Maybe you became your mother's therapist or your father's emotional spouse. Maybe you learned to suppress your own needs because there was 'already too much going on' and your problems would just add to the burden.

Parentified children learn that their value comes from taking care of others. That their needs don't matter as much as everyone else's. That love is something you earn through service, not something you receive simply for existing.

As adults, parentified children become the person everyone calls in a crisis but who never calls anyone themselves. They become the partner who does all the emotional labour. The employee who takes on everyone's work. The friend who's always available but never asks for support.

They're exhausted. Always. Because they never learned to stop. They never learned that they don't have to earn love through caretaking. They never learned that it's okay to need help too.

If you were parentified, you probably have a deeply ingrained belief that asking for help is weakness. That your needs are burdensome. That you should be able to handle everything yourself. These aren't truths. They're trauma responses.

You were a child forced to be an adult. You didn't fail at childhood. Childhood failed you. And now you get to learn what you should have learned then: that you matter. That your needs are legitimate. That you're allowed to receive, not just give.

The Good Child Syndrome

The 'good child' is the one who never caused problems. Never talked back. Always got good grades. Made the parents look good. Was responsible, mature, 'easy.'

Sounds great, right? Here's what nobody tells you: being the 'good child' is exhausting. And it's a setup for a lifetime of self-abandonment.

Good children learn to read what others need and become that. They develop an exquisite sensitivity to other people's emotional states and a complete blindness to their own. They achieve and perform and accommodate until they don't know who they are underneath all that compliance.

As adults, former good children are often the ones who:

- Can't say no without feeling guilty
- Struggle to identify what they actually want
- Feel responsible for everyone's happiness
- Experience success but never feel successful
- Burn out repeatedly because they can't stop performing
- Get praised for being 'low-maintenance' while slowly dying inside
- Have a deep fear of disappointing people
- Struggle with perfectionism and shame

If you were the good child, you learned that your authentic self wasn't acceptable. That love required constant performance. That making waves, having needs, or disappointing people was unacceptable. You learned to perform 'good' instead of being real.

And now you're an adult who's terrified of being 'too much' or 'not enough.' You're constantly adjusting yourself to fit what you think others want. You're exhausted from performing. And you have no idea who you actually are underneath all those masks.

The good news? You can stop performing. You can discover who you are when you're not trying to be what everyone else needs. But it requires making people uncomfortable. It requires disappointing them sometimes. It requires being 'difficult.'

And that feels impossible. Because your whole identity is built on being easy, accommodating, low-maintenance.

But that's not a real identity. That's just a survival strategy that outlived its usefulness.

The Scapegoat's Burden

While the good child was earning love through compliance, the scapegoat was blamed for everything. Every family problem, every parental frustration, every bit of dysfunction got projected onto this one kid.

Scapegoats learn different lessons about self-betrayal. They learn that they're fundamentally flawed. That no matter what they do, it will be wrong. That they deserve poor treatment. That rebellion is the only form of autonomy available to them.

The scapegoat's version of self-betrayal looks different from the good child's, but it's just as damaging. They learned that they're not worthy of good treatment, so they accept crumbs. They learned that they're the problem, so they don't set boundaries because 'who are they to ask for better?'

As adults, former scapegoats often:

- Struggle with deep shame and low self-worth
- Expect rejection and sabotage good things before they can be hurt
- Have a hard time trusting that people actually care
- Swing between isolation and intense enmeshment
- Self-sabotage when things are going well
- Struggle to believe they deserve better
- Have a high tolerance for mistreatment

If you were the scapegoat, you internalized the message that you're inherently bad, wrong, too much, not enough.

And now you unconsciously seek out relationships that confirm that belief. You attract people who treat you poorly because that feels familiar. That feels like home.

And here's the cruel irony: when someone treats you well, it feels wrong. Uncomfortable. Suspicious. So you push them away or sabotage the relationship because kindness doesn't match your internal programming about what you deserve.

Breaking this pattern requires challenging your core belief about yourself. It requires recognizing that you weren't the problem. The family system was. It requires learning that you deserve kindness, respect, and good treatment. Not because you've earned it. Just because you exist.

The Lost Child

There's another role that gets less attention but is just as damaging: the lost child. The one who learned to disappear. Who stayed quiet, stayed out of the way, didn't ask for anything, didn't cause any trouble.

Lost children learned that the safest strategy was invisibility. That their needs didn't matter. That they could avoid pain by not having expectations. So they became experts at not needing anything from anyone.

As adults, former lost children:

- Struggle to ask for help or support
- Feel invisible in relationships
- Have difficulty identifying their own needs
- Minimize their pain and problems
- Feel like they don't matter

- Struggle with feeling lonely even in relationships
- Have a hard time taking up space

If you were the lost child, you learned that you don't matter. That your presence is neutral at best, burdensome at worst. That the best you can hope for is to not be a problem. So you made yourself small. You learned to need nothing. You perfected the art of invisibility.

And now you're an adult who people overlook. Who gets forgotten about. Who doesn't get invited. Not because you're unlovable, but because you've trained everyone in your life that you don't need anything, so they don't think to include you.

Unlearning this requires the opposite of what you learned: it requires making yourself visible. It requires asking for things. It requires believing that you matter enough to take up space.

The Patterns You're Repeating

Here's the thing about childhood programming: you'll keep repeating it until you become conscious of it. You'll choose partners who treat you the way your parents did. You'll create work environments that mirror your family dynamics. You'll find friends who expect the same self-abandonment you learned at home.

It's not because you're stupid or broken. It's because familiar feels like home, even when home was dysfunctional. Your nervous system learned early that this is what relationships look like. This is what love feels like. This is your role.

And until you unlearn it, you'll keep casting yourself in the same role in different productions. Different setting, different actors, same script.

Examples of how patterns repeat:

• The parentified child becomes the partner who manages all the emotional labour while their spouse contributes nothing

• The good child becomes the employee who can't say no and gets exploited by their boss

• The scapegoat attracts friends who blame them for everything that goes wrong

• The lost child ends up in relationships where they feel invisible and unimportant

You're not choosing these situations consciously. You're unconsciously recreating your childhood dynamics because that's what your nervous system knows. That's what feels normal.

But normal doesn't mean healthy. And familiar doesn't mean good. It just means you've done it before.

How the Patterns Show Up Now

Let's get specific about how childhood programming manifests in adult life:

In romantic relationships: You choose partners who are emotionally unavailable (like your distant parent), or demanding and critical (like your controlling parent), or unstable (like your unpredictable parent). You recreate the dynamic you learned, hoping this time you'll finally earn the love you couldn't get as a child.

At work: You take on way too much because you learned your worth is tied to productivity. You can't set boundaries with your boss because authority figures are scary. You work yourself to exhaustion trying to prove you're valuable.

With friends: You're always the one giving support but never asking for it. You're the therapist friend. The one who everyone calls in a crisis. But when you need help? Silence. Because you never learned how to receive.

With yourself: You're your own worst critic. You talk to yourself in ways you'd never talk to anyone else. You hold yourself to impossible standards. You punish yourself for being human. Because that's how you were treated, so that's how you learned to treat yourself.

The patterns are everywhere once you start looking for them. And seeing them clearly is the first step to changing them.

The Cultural and Gender Dimensions

Your family wasn't operating in a vacuum. They were influenced by cultural norms, gender expectations, and societal conditioning.

If you're a woman or femme-presenting, you were likely taught that your value lies in being nurturing, accommodating, and selfless. That taking care of others is your highest calling. That having needs makes you selfish. That boundaries make you difficult.

If you're a man or mask-presenting, you were likely taught to suppress emotions, avoid vulnerability, and maintain control at all costs. That asking for help is weakness. That emotions are for women. That your worth is tied to your achievements and ability to provide.

These gendered messages compound family dysfunction. They make it even harder to recognize self-betrayal because it's packaged as virtue. Women are praised for self-sacrifice. Men are praised for emotional stoicism. Both are forms of self-abandonment, just differently packaged.

Cultural background matters too. Some cultures emphasize collectivism over individualism. Family needs over personal needs. This can be beautiful. It can also be weaponized to guilt you into accepting dysfunction.

Honouring your culture doesn't mean accepting abuse. Respecting your elders doesn't mean tolerating disrespect. You can maintain cultural values while also maintaining boundaries.

The Way Out

The way out starts with awareness. With recognizing that the lessons you learned weren't truth. They were survival strategies that made sense in context but don't serve you anymore.

You don't have to keep performing. You don't have to keep shrinking. You don't have to keep managing everyone else's emotions while ignoring your own. You don't have to keep earning love through service. You don't have to keep accepting crumbs.

You can learn new patterns. You can practice self-honouring even when it feels uncomfortable. You can choose differently even when the old programming screams at you that you're being selfish, difficult, or wrong.

This is the work. Not just understanding where it came from, but actively choosing something different. Over and over. Until the new pattern becomes as automatic as the old one used to be.

Here's what that looks like practically:

- Notice when you're abandoning yourself in real-time
- Name the pattern: 'This is my good child programming. This is my parentified child response.'
- Pause before automatically complying
- Ask yourself: What do I actually want here? What would honouring myself look like?
- Choose differently, even if it feels terrifying
- Tolerate the discomfort of disappointing people
- Repeat until it gets easier

You're not doomed to repeat your family's dysfunction. But you do have to do the work of unlearning it. You have to be willing to see the patterns clearly, understand where they came from, and consciously choose something different.

This isn't about blaming your parents. This isn't about playing victim. This is about taking responsibility for your own healing. About recognizing that what you learned then doesn't have to define you now.

You get to write a new script. You get to break the cycle. You get to be the generation that chooses differently.

But first, you have to see the old script clearly. You have to understand the programming. You have to recognize when it's running.

That's what this chapter is about. Seeing it. Naming it. Understanding it. So you can finally let it go.

PART TWO:
FAMILY DYNAMICS

Chapter 4: It's Okay If They Don't Like Your Boundaries

Let's get something straight right now: your family will not throw you a parade when you start setting boundaries. They will not celebrate your newfound self-respect. They will not say, 'We're so proud of you for finally standing up for yourself!'

They're going to be pissed.

And that's okay. Actually, it's more than okay. It's expected. People who benefited from your lack of boundaries are rarely thrilled when you install some. It disrupts the system. It changes the dynamic. It means they have to adjust.

Tough.

Your family's comfort is not more important than your wellbeing. Their approval is not worth your sanity. Their disappointment is not your emergency.

This chapter is about giving you permission to set boundaries with family even when, especially when, they don't like it.

Why Family Boundaries Feel Impossible

Family is where most people's boundary muscles are weakest. You can set boundaries at work. You can set them with friends. You can even set them with strangers.

But family? That's where all the programming kicks in hardest.

Because with family, there's history. There's obligation. There's this idea that blood relations come with unlimited access passes. There's the fear that boundaries equal rejection. That saying no to your mother means you don't love her. That protecting yourself from your father's criticism means you're ungrateful.

Plus, your family knows all your buttons, because they installed most of them. They know exactly how to make you feel guilty. They know your weak spots. They've had years, decades even, to perfect the art of getting you to cave.

They know what works. 'After everything I've done for you...' 'Family is supposed to be there for each other.' 'You've changed.' 'Why are you being so sensitive?'

These aren't just random comments. These are precision-guided guilt missiles, designed to hit exactly where you're most vulnerable.

And here's the other reason family boundaries feel impossible: you were literally raised by these people. Their voices are in your head. Their judgments shaped your sense of self. Disappointing them feels like betraying your own identity.

But here's the truth: setting boundaries with family isn't betrayal. It's evolution. It's growing up. It's recognizing that the rules that governed your childhood don't have to govern your adult life.

The Guilt Trip Playbook

Let's talk about the greatest hits of family guilt trips. Because if you can recognize them, they lose some of their power.

'After everything I've done for you...' Translation: You owe me unlimited compliance because I performed basic parental duties.

Nope. Parents are supposed to take care of their kids. That's the deal. You don't owe them your entire adult life in exchange for being fed and clothed as a child. You didn't ask to be born. They chose to have you. Your existence is not a debt.

Yes, you can be grateful for what they provided. But gratitude doesn't mean you surrender your autonomy. Appreciation doesn't mean you accept disrespect. Thankfulness doesn't mean you have no boundaries.

When someone uses 'after everything I've done for you' as leverage, they're not asking you to be grateful. They're demanding compliance. Big difference.

'Family is supposed to be there for each other.' Translation: You're supposed to be there for me, specifically, in whatever way I demand, regardless of your own needs.

Yes, healthy families support each other. Mutually. Reciprocally. Not one person doing all the giving while everyone else does all the taking. 'Being there' doesn't mean abandoning your own wellbeing to manage someone else's dysfunction.

Being there for family can look like: listening when they need to talk, helping when you're able, showing up for important events. Being there does NOT mean:

accepting abuse, tolerating disrespect, sacrificing your mental health, being available 24/7, or doing everything they ask.

Real family support goes both ways. If they're not there for you the way you're there for them, that's not family. That's exploitation.

'You've changed.' Translation: You're not as easy to control anymore and I don't like it.

Yes, you have changed. You've developed self-respect. You've learned to honour your needs. You've stopped accepting poor treatment. That's called growth. The fact that they're framing it as a problem tells you everything you need to know.

When someone says 'you've changed' as an accusation, what they mean is: 'You used to do what I wanted, and now you don't, and I'm uncomfortable with that.'

Your response? 'Yes, I have changed. I've learned to respect myself.' Then stop explaining. You don't owe anyone a defence of your personal growth.

'Why are you being so sensitive/dramatic/difficult?' Translation: Your needs inconvenience me and I'd like you to go back to having none.

Asking to be treated with basic respect is not being dramatic. Setting boundaries is not being difficult. Refusing to tolerate dysfunction is not being sensitive. These are manipulation tactics designed to make you second-guess your reality.

When someone calls you 'too sensitive' for having boundaries, they're really saying you're not letting them treat you poorly anymore and they're annoyed about it.

Here's a test: if your boundary is 'please don't yell at me,' and their response is 'you're being too sensitive,' the problem isn't your sensitivity. The problem is their yelling.

'I'm your mother/father.' Translation: My parental status entitles me to unlimited access and zero accountability.

Being someone's parent doesn't exempt you from treating them with respect. It doesn't grant immunity from boundaries. It doesn't mean you get to say or do whatever you want without consequences.

Yes, they're your parent. And you're their adult child, which means you're an autonomous person with the right to set boundaries about how you're treated.

Respect goes both ways. Always.

The Extinction Burst

Here's what happens when you first start enforcing boundaries with family: things get worse before they get better. Way worse.

This is called an extinction burst in psychology. When a behaviour that used to work (guilt-tripping you, boundary-testing, emotional manipulation) suddenly stops working, people escalate. They turn up the volume. They get more dramatic. They pull out all the stops.

Think of it like a vending machine. If you put money in and press a button, you expect a snack. But if the machine stops working, what do you do? You don't just walk away. First, you press the button harder. Then you press it multiple times. Then you shake the machine. Then you kick it. You escalate your efforts to get the result you're used to getting.

That's what family does when boundaries are new. They escalate. They cry harder. They rage louder. They guilt-trip more intensely. They threaten more dramatically.

They're not doing this because your boundaries are wrong. They're doing it because boundaries are new and uncomfortable and they're hoping if they make enough noise, you'll cave and go back to the old system.

This is where most people give up. This is where you say, 'See? Setting boundaries just makes everything worse. It's easier to just go back to the way things were.'

Don't.

The extinction burst is temporary. It's a test. If you hold firm, it stops. They learn that escalation doesn't work anymore. They adjust to the new reality.

But if you cave during the extinction burst, you've just taught them that if they make enough noise, you'll fold. And guess what they'll do next time? Make even more noise. Because it worked.

Hold the line. Let them be upset. Let them escalate. Let them have their feelings about your boundaries. And keep enforcing them anyway.

Eventually, they'll adjust. Or they won't. Either way, you'll have protected yourself.

The 'But They're Family' Trap

'But they're family' is one of the most toxic phrases in the English language. It's used to justify abuse, excuse dysfunction, and guilt people into tolerating behaviour they would never accept from anyone else.

You know what being family actually means? It means you had the bad luck to be born into the same gene pool. That's it. It doesn't mean you owe them unlimited access to your life, your time, your energy, or your sanity.

Being family doesn't exempt people from treating you with basic respect. Being family doesn't mean boundaries don't apply. Being family doesn't mean you have to tolerate toxic behaviour, emotional manipulation, or consistent disrespect.

If anything, family should be held to higher standards, not lower ones. These are the people who are supposed to love you most. If they can't manage basic human decency, why exactly are you protecting them from consequences?

Here's a thought experiment: if a stranger, coworker, or acquaintance treated you the way your family member treats you, would you tolerate it? Would you make excuses for it? Would you keep going back for more?

No. You'd cut them off immediately. You'd recognize it as toxic. You'd protect yourself.

But because it's family, you tolerate it. You make excuses. You minimize the impact. You tell yourself it's not that bad.

Stop. Being related to someone doesn't make their bad behaviour acceptable. Shared DNA doesn't grant immunity from consequences.

You can love someone and still protect yourself from them. You can be family and still have boundaries. You can honour the relationship without accepting the abuse.

What Good Family Boundaries Look Like

Good family boundaries aren't walls that shut everyone out. They're clear lines that protect your wellbeing while still allowing connection, if the other person is willing to respect them.

Here are examples of healthy family boundaries:

- 'I'm happy to visit, but we're leaving at 8pm.' (Time boundaries)
- 'I love you, but I'm not discussing my relationship/job/life choices with you.' (Topic boundaries)
- 'You're welcome in my home, but if you criticize me/my partner/my parenting, the visit ends.' (Behavioural boundaries)
- 'I'll help when I can, but I'm not available every time you call with an emergency.' (Availability boundaries)
- 'That topic isn't up for discussion.' (Conversation boundaries)
- 'I need 24 hours' notice before visits.' (Space boundaries)
- 'I don't respond to texts/calls after 9pm.' (Communication boundaries)

Notice what these have in common? They're clear. They're non-negotiable. They specify both what you will do and what you won't do. And they don't require the other person's approval or understanding.

Good boundaries also include consequences. 'If you continue to [behaviour], I will [consequence].' And then you actually follow through.

Examples with consequences:

- 'If you raise your voice at me, I'm ending this conversation.'
- 'If you bring up my weight again, I'm leaving.'
- 'If you can't respect my parenting choices, you won't have unsupervised time with my kids.'
- 'If you show up unannounced again, I won't answer the door.'

The consequence has to be something you're actually willing and able to enforce. Don't threaten to cut off all contact if you're not prepared to do that. Don't threaten to leave if you have no way to leave.

Start with boundaries you can hold. Build from there.

Common Boundary Violations (And How to Handle Them)

Let's get specific about the boundary violations that happen most often with family:

The Drop-In: They show up unannounced and expect you to accommodate them.

Response: Don't answer the door. Or answer and say, 'I'm not available right now. Please call ahead next time.' Then close the door.

They'll be offended. Let them. Showing up unannounced is disrespectful of your time and space. You're not being rude by enforcing this boundary. They're being rude by violating it.

The Interrogation: They ask invasive questions about your life, finances, relationships, or choices.

Response: 'I'm not discussing that.' Repeat as necessary. Don't JADE (Justify, Argue, Defend, Explain). The more you explain why you won't discuss it, the more ammunition you give them.

The Guilt Trip: 'I guess I'm just a terrible mother.' 'Fine, I'll just die alone then.' 'After everything I've done...'

Response: 'I hear that you're upset. My boundary stands.' Don't argue with their feelings. Don't try to convince them they're not a terrible mother. Don't fall for the manipulation.

The Triangulation: They talk about you to other family members to recruit allies against your boundaries.

Response: 'If you have an issue with me, please discuss it with me directly.' And to the flying monkeys they send: 'This is between me and [person]. I'm not discussing it with you.'

The Silent Treatment: They punish your boundaries by withdrawing, ignoring you, or freezing you out.

Response: Nothing. Let them have their tantrum. The silent treatment is emotional abuse designed to make you so uncomfortable that you'll abandon your boundary to make it stop. Don't. Use the silence to rest. Enjoy the peace. They'll come back when they realize it's not working.

The Boundary Testing: They 'forget' your boundary or claim they 'didn't know' to see if you'll enforce it.

Response: Enforce it immediately. 'As I mentioned, I don't discuss that topic. Let's talk about something else or I'm going to end this call.' Then follow through if they continue.

Dealing With the Fallout

When you set boundaries, some family members will respect them. Some will push back but eventually adjust. And some will refuse to adapt and may distance themselves or escalate their behaviour.

That third group is painful. But it's also important information. Someone who would rather end the relationship than treat you with respect is telling you exactly how conditional their love really was.

And that hurts. Of course it does. You wanted them to love you enough to change. You wanted them to value the relationship more than their need for control. You wanted them to choose connection over ego.

But they didn't. And that's on them, not you.

Your boundaries didn't ruin the relationship. Your boundaries revealed what kind of relationship it actually was. There's a difference.

The people who truly love you will adjust. They might not like the boundaries at first. They might push back. They might need time to accept the new dynamic. But ultimately, they'll respect your boundaries because they care about the relationship more than they care about control.

The ones who can't adjust? They were never loving you. They were using you. And discovering that is painful but also liberating. Because now you know. Now you can stop wasting energy on people who were never going to give you what you need.

Your Script for Boundary Enforcement

Here are scripts you can use when family pushes back on your boundaries:

When they test the boundary: 'I understand you're disappointed. The boundary stands.'

Don't apologize for the boundary. Don't over-explain. Don't negotiate. Just restate it calmly and move on.

When they ask why: 'Because it doesn't work for me.'

You don't owe anyone a detailed explanation of why you have the boundaries you have. 'It doesn't work for me' is a complete sentence.

When they guilt trip: 'I hear that you're upset. I'm still not changing my mind.'

Acknowledge their feelings without changing your boundary. Their feelings are valid. Your boundary is also valid. Both can be true.

When they escalate: 'I'm going to go now. We can talk when you're ready to be respectful.'

Then actually leave/end the call/stop responding. Don't keep engaging with someone who's yelling, insulting, or manipulating. Remove yourself from the situation.

When they bring up the past: 'I'm not discussing the past. I'm setting a boundary for the present.'

Don't get pulled into relitigating old grievances. Stay focused on the current boundary.

When they cry: 'I can see this is hard for you. I'm still holding this boundary.'

Tears are a manipulation tactic for some people. Don't let crying override your boundary. You can be compassionate about their feelings while still protecting yourself.

When Boundaries Mean Distance

Sometimes, the only way to maintain boundaries with family is to create physical or emotional distance. This might look like:

- Reducing the frequency of visits
- Keeping phone calls short and surface-level
- Only seeing them in public places or with other people present
- Taking breaks from contact when they violate boundaries
- Limiting what personal information you share

This isn't punishment. This is protection. You're creating the conditions under which you can maintain a relationship without sacrificing your wellbeing.

And if they can't respect even these modified boundaries? Then you might need to consider very low contact or no contact. That's a last resort, but sometimes it's the only option that protects your mental health.

The Permission You're Waiting For

You don't need your family's permission to set boundaries. You don't need them to agree that the boundaries are reasonable. You don't need them to understand why the boundaries are necessary.

You just need to set them. And enforce them. And live with the discomfort of their disappointment while protecting your own wellbeing.

Here's your permission: It's okay if they don't like your boundaries. It's okay if they're upset. It's okay if they think you've changed. It's okay if they complain to other family members about you. It's okay if they give you the silent treatment.

Their reaction is their problem to manage. Your job is to hold the boundary.

You are not responsible for managing their emotions about your boundaries. You are not required to shrink yourself to make them comfortable. You are not obligated to accept disrespect because 'that's just how they are.'

They raised you. You love them (maybe). You're grateful for what they've given you (hopefully). And none of that means you have to accept less than basic respect.

You can honour your family without dishonouring yourself. You can maintain relationships without sacrificing your sanity. You can set boundaries and still love them.

But you cannot set boundaries and expect everyone to be happy about it. And that's okay.

Their happiness with your boundaries is not required for the boundaries to be valid. Your wellbeing is not negotiable. Your peace is not up for debate. So set the boundaries. Enforce them. And let your family have their feelings about it. It's okay if they don't like your boundaries. Really. It's okay.

Chapter 5: You Can Honor Your Parents Without Dishonouring Yourself

Here's the lie you've been fed: honouring your parents means doing whatever they want, whenever they want it, regardless of how it affects you. It means never saying no, never setting boundaries, and never prioritizing your own needs over their expectations.

That's not honour. That's servitude.

Real honour looks different. Real honour means treating your parents with respect while also respecting yourself. It means appreciating what they've given you while not accepting what they're taking from you. It means loving them without losing yourself.

This chapter is about finding that balance. About maintaining a relationship with your parents (if you choose to) without sacrificing your own wellbeing in the process.

What You Actually Owe Your Parents

Let's clear this up once and for all: what do you actually owe your parents?

Basic respect? Sure. Appreciation for the things they did right? Absolutely. Your entire adult life arranged around their comfort and expectations? No.

Here's what you don't owe them:

- A specific career path they chose for you
- A specific relationship status or partner they approve of
- Grandchildren on their timeline (or at all)

- Daily phone calls or constant availability
- Unlimited emotional support while they provide none
- Agreement with all their opinions and values
- Tolerance of disrespect or abuse
- Abandonment of your own dreams and goals
- Your mental health and peace of mind
- A relationship if they're consistently harmful

Parenting is not a transaction where children owe their parents payback for being raised. Your parents made a choice to have you. That came with responsibilities. Meeting those responsibilities doesn't create a debt that you spend your whole life repaying.

You didn't sign a contract when you were born that said, 'I agree to live my life according to your specifications in exchange for being raised.' They chose to have a child. They chose to take on the responsibilities that come with that. You don't owe them your autonomy as payment.

Now, does this mean you should be ungrateful or dismissive of what they've done for you? Of course not. Gratitude is important. Appreciation is valuable. But gratitude doesn't equal obligation to accept poor treatment. Appreciation doesn't mean surrendering your right to boundaries.

You can be thankful for the good while also protecting yourself from the bad. Both things can be true at the same time.

The Cultural Weight of Parental Obligation

Different cultures have different expectations about what children owe their parents. Some cultures emphasize independence, you're expected to go off and build your own life. Others emphasize filial duty, you're expected to prioritize parental needs throughout your life.

If you come from a culture with strong filial piety traditions, setting boundaries with parents might feel like cultural betrayal. Like you're abandoning your heritage, your values, everything you were raised to believe was right.

You might hear: 'This isn't how we do things in our culture.' 'You're becoming too Western.' 'You've forgotten where you came from.' 'This is disrespectful to our traditions.'

And that hits different than regular guilt trips. Because it's not just about disappointing your parents. It's about betraying your entire cultural identity. It's about being labelled as someone who's lost their way, forgotten their roots, abandoned their people.

But here's the thing: honouring your culture doesn't mean accepting dysfunction. Respecting tradition doesn't mean tolerating abuse. Your culture's beautiful emphasis on family connection shouldn't be weaponized to guilt you into accepting treatment that harms you.

Every culture has both beauty and dysfunction. You get to keep the beautiful parts, the emphasis on family, the respect for elders, the value of community, while also rejecting the parts that don't serve you. The parts that demand you sacrifice your wellbeing. The parts that prioritize obedience over health. The parts that confuse control with care.

You can maintain cultural values while also maintaining boundaries. You can honour the good parts of your upbringing while rejecting the harmful parts. This isn't cultural betrayal. It's cultural evolution.

You're not abandoning your culture. You're adapting it. You're taking what works and releasing what doesn't. That's not disrespectful. That's wisdom.

The Special Challenge of Immigrant Parents

If your parents are immigrants, whether to another city country or culture, there's often an extra layer of guilt. They sacrificed everything to give you opportunities. They left their home, their family, their entire life behind. They worked jobs beneath their qualifications. They endured discrimination. They struggled so you wouldn't have to.

And that sacrifice is real. That struggle is real. That deserves acknowledgment and gratitude.

But it still doesn't mean you owe them your entire life.

Their sacrifice was their choice. They made it hoping you'd have a better life. But 'better life' doesn't mean 'a life arranged entirely around making us comfortable.' It doesn't mean you can never disappoint them. It doesn't mean you have to live the exact life they envisioned for you.

You can honour their sacrifice by living well, by being successful in your own way, by appreciating what they gave you. You don't honour their sacrifice by destroying yourself to meet their expectations.

They didn't sacrifice everything so you could sacrifice yourself. They sacrificed so you could have freedom, opportunity, choice. Use it.

When Your Parents Are Toxic

Not all parents deserve unconditional access to their adult children. Some parents are genuinely toxic. Abusive. Manipulative. Narcissistic. Unwilling to change or take accountability for the harm they've caused.

And if that's your situation, you're allowed to protect yourself. Even from them. Especially from them.

'But they did their best' doesn't erase harm. Their best might have been terrible. Their best might have been abusive. Their best might have left you with trauma that you'll spend years healing from.

Intention doesn't cancel impact. Maybe they didn't mean to hurt you. Maybe they were doing what was done to them. Maybe they were struggling with their own unhealed wounds. All of that can be true. They simply didn't know better. But you can still need to protect yourself from them even if you forgive them.

You can acknowledge that your parents had their own trauma while also acknowledging that they hurt you. Both things can be true. Their pain explains their behaviour-it doesn't condone it.

Here are signs your parent might be toxic:

• They refuse to respect your boundaries no matter how clearly you state them

• They use guilt and manipulation as their primary communication style

• They make everything about them, even your accomplishments or struggles

• They undermine your confidence and self-worth consistently

• They refuse to take accountability for their behaviour

• They turn family members against you when you set boundaries

• They punish you emotionally for not complying with their wishes

• They violate your privacy, autonomy, or personal space repeatedly

• They use your vulnerabilities against you

• They create drama and chaos that you're expected to fix

If multiple items on that list sound familiar, you might have a toxic parent. And that's not your fault. You didn't cause their toxicity. You can't cure it. And you don't have to accept it.

The Different Levels of Contact

Boundaries with parents exist on a spectrum. You get to choose where on that spectrum works for you. There's no universal 'right' answer. There's only what protects your wellbeing while maintaining whatever level of connection you're comfortable with.

Full contact: Regular interaction with healthy boundaries in place. You see them often, but on your terms, with clear limits about what's acceptable.

This works when your parents are generally healthy people who respect boundaries even if they don't always like them. You can maintain frequent contact because they don't consistently violate your limits. You have regular visits, phone calls, involvement in each other's lives. With clear rules about what topics are off-limits, what behaviour isn't acceptable, and what consequences exist for violations.

Reduced contact: Less frequent interaction. You see them for holidays, special occasions, but not regularly. You limit the topics you'll discuss. You keep visits short.

This works when your parents aren't respectful enough for full contact but aren't harmful enough to cut off entirely. You maintain the relationship but with significant limitations. Maybe you see them a few times a year instead of weekly. Maybe you keep phone calls to ten minutes instead of an hour. Maybe you only see them in public places or with other people present.

Low contact: Minimal interaction. Occasional phone calls. Holiday cards. You maintain the connection but from a distance that feels safe.

This works when direct contact is too stressful but you're not ready to completely sever ties. Maybe you text on birthdays. Maybe you send a holiday card. Maybe you attend family events once a year. You're technically still in contact, but barely. You've created maximum distance while maintaining a thread of connection.

No contact: Complete cessation of relationship. This is the nuclear option, but sometimes it's the only option that protects your wellbeing.

This is appropriate when your parents are so consistently harmful that any contact damages your mental health. When they refuse to respect any boundary. When contact with them triggers your trauma responses. When the relationship is purely destructive with no redeeming value.

No contact is not failure. It's not cruel. It's not ungrateful. It's survival. It's recognizing that some relationships are so toxic that the only way to protect yourself is to end them entirely.

You're allowed to choose any of these options. Your mental health, your safety, your peace matter more than anyone else's opinion about what you 'should' do.

The Guilt of Choosing Distance

If you've chosen reduced contact, low contact, or no contact with your parents, you probably feel guilty. Intensely guilty. Like you're failing some fundamental duty. Like you're a bad person.

You're not.

Choosing distance from parents who harm you isn't cruel. It's self-preservation. It's recognizing that the relationship as it exists is damaging and choosing to protect yourself.

The guilt you feel? That's old programming. That's years of being told that family is everything, that you owe your parents unconditional access, that 'honouring your parents' means tolerating whatever they dish out.

But here's the truth: you can honour your parents by living well, by healing from what they did, by breaking the cycle so you don't repeat their mistakes. You don't honour them by letting them continue to harm you.

If you feel guilty for protecting yourself from your parents, ask yourself: would you tell a friend to maintain contact with someone who treats them the way your parents treat you? Would you tell them they're obligated to keep accepting that treatment because 'that's just how they are'?

No. You'd tell them to protect themselves. You'd support their decision to create distance. You'd validate that they deserve better.

Give yourself the same compassion you'd give a friend.

Setting Boundaries Without Guilt (Or: How to Feel Guilty and Do It Anyway)

Here's the secret: you're probably going to feel guilty when you set boundaries with your parents. The guilt is normal. It's expected. It's part of the process.

The goal isn't to eliminate the guilt. The goal is to act in alignment with your values despite the guilt.

You can love your parents and still set boundaries. You can appreciate what they've given you and still refuse what they're taking. You can honour them and still respect yourself.

In fact, setting healthy boundaries with your parents is one of the most respectful things you can do. It says: 'I value our relationship enough to want it to be healthy. I care about us enough to be honest about what I can and can't accept. I respect you enough to tell you the truth instead of lying and resenting you.'

The parents who love you will eventually hear that. They might not like the boundaries initially. They might push back. They might need time to adjust. But if they genuinely care about the relationship, they'll work to respect your limits.

The ones who can't? They're telling you that control matters more to them than connection. That their comfort matters more than your wellbeing. That they'd rather lose the relationship than respect your autonomy.

And that's painful information to receive. But it's also liberating. Because now you know where you stand.

Navigating the Practical Realities

Setting boundaries with aging parents gets complicated. What if they need care? What if they're sick? What if you're the only child who can help? What about guilt? What about duty? What about the fact that someday they'll be gone and you don't want to have regrets?

These are real concerns. And the answer isn't 'abandon them to suffer.' The answer is: 'You can help within the limits of what's sustainable for you.'

You can assist with practical needs while maintaining emotional boundaries. You can hire help instead of being the help. You can coordinate care without being the primary caregiver. You can contribute financially without contributing your entire life. You can help them find resources without being the resource.

Helping your parents doesn't require self-sacrifice. You can support them while also supporting yourself. That's not selfish. That's sustainable.

Here are ways to help aging parents while maintaining boundaries:

- Research and arrange for professional caregivers instead of doing all the care yourself
- Coordinate care among siblings or other family members instead of shouldering it alone
- Set specific times/days when you're available to help instead of being on-call 24/7
- Hire someone to handle tasks you find particularly draining
- Set up systems and services that reduce hands-on involvement

• Attend doctor appointments but maintain boundaries around other topics

• Help with logistics while limiting emotional engagement

Your parents' needs are real. Your limits are also real. Finding the overlap between what they need and what you can sustainably provide is the goal.

And if they refuse help from anyone but you? That's a choice they're making. That's manipulation. You're not obligated to be the only acceptable help. You can offer alternatives. If they reject those alternatives, that's on them.

The 'Someday They'll Be Gone' Guilt

'Someday they'll be gone and you'll regret this.' 'You only get one mother/father.' 'You'll wish you'd tried harder when it's too late.'

This is one of the most powerful guilt trips because it might be true. Your parents will die someday. And you might feel regret.

But here's what that guilt trip doesn't mention: you'll also regret sacrificing years of your life trying to fix an unfixable relationship. You'll regret the toll it took on your mental health. You'll regret the opportunities you missed because you were too drained from managing their dysfunction.

Regret exists on both sides of this choice. You might regret creating distance. You might also regret not creating it sooner. The question isn't 'which choice has zero regret?' The question is 'which choice protects my wellbeing?'

And here's another truth: trying harder doesn't fix toxic relationships. You could give everything, your time, your energy, your mental health, your entire life, and it still wouldn't be enough. Because the problem isn't that you're not trying hard enough. The problem is that they're not healthy enough to have a healthy relationship with.

You can't love someone into being different. You can't sacrifice yourself into making them change. You can't accommodate them into respecting you without boundaries.

So yes, someday they'll be gone. And you might feel regret. But you'll feel less regret if you protected yourself than if you destroyed yourself trying to fix what was never yours to fix.

When They Cry

One of the hardest things about setting boundaries with parents is watching them cry. Seeing them hurt. Knowing you're the cause of their pain.

Here's what you need to remember: you're not causing their pain. Their inability to respect your boundaries is causing their pain. Their attachment to control is causing their pain. Their refusal to accept that you're an autonomous adult is causing their pain.

You're not being cruel by having boundaries. You're being healthy. Their tears don't make your boundaries invalid. Their sadness doesn't mean you're wrong.

You can be compassionate about their feelings while still maintaining your boundary. 'I can see this is hard for you. I'm still not changing my decision.'

Let them cry. Let them be sad. Let them grieve the version of you that did whatever they wanted. That version wasn't real anyway. It was you performing. They're not losing you. They're losing their unlimited access to you. There's a difference.

Honouring Them Through Living Well

Here's a radical thought: maybe the best way to honour your parents is to live well. To heal from what they did. To build a life that doesn't repeat their mistakes. To be happy, healthy, and whole.

Maybe honouring them doesn't look like compliance. Maybe it looks like becoming the person you couldn't be when you were busy managing their emotions and meeting their expectations.

Maybe the greatest tribute to their sacrifice (if they sacrificed) is using the opportunities they gave you to build a genuinely good life. Not the life they wanted for you. The life that actually makes you happy.

You honour your parents by:

- Breaking generational cycles of dysfunction
- Healing your trauma so you don't pass it on
- Building healthy relationships based on respect, not control
- Living authentically instead of performing
- Creating a life that brings you genuine joy
- Becoming the parent you needed (if you choose to have children)
- Refusing to repeat their mistakes

That's honour. Real honour. Not servitude. Not self-abandonment. Not compliance.

Living well, being healthy, choosing yourself. That honours them more than destroying yourself ever could.

The Permission You Don't Need

You don't need your parents' permission to:

- Live where you want
- Pursue the career you want
- Marry (or not marry) who you want
- Have (or not have) children
- Make your own choices about your own life
- Set boundaries that protect your wellbeing
- Choose reduced or no contact if necessary
- Heal from what they did
- Be different from them
- Prioritize your own happiness

Their approval would be nice. Of course it would. But it's not required. And waiting for permission to live your life on your own terms is a waste of your one precious life.

You're an adult. You get to make adult decisions. And one of those decisions is how much access your parents have to you and your life.

You can honour your parents without dishonouring yourself. You can love them without losing yourself. You can appreciate what they've given you without accepting what they're taking from you.

But you have to believe that you're allowed to do that. You have to believe that your wellbeing matters as much as their comfort. You have to believe that boundaries aren't betrayal.

So, here's your permission, one more time: It's okay to set boundaries with your parents. It's okay if they don't like it. It's okay if they cry. It's okay if they're disappointed. It's okay if they think you've changed.

You can love them and love yourself. Both things can be true.

Chapter 6: Their Expectations Are Not Your Emergency

Your mother expected you to call daily. Your father expected you to take over the family business. Your aunt expected you to give her grandkids by 30. Your whole family expected you to stay local, marry the right person, choose the right career, live the right life.

Their expectations. Not yours.

Here's what nobody tells you: other people's expectations of you are their problem, not yours. Their disappointment is theirs to manage. Their unmet expectations are not your failure.

You didn't sign up for the life they planned for you. You don't owe anyone the fulfilment of their fantasies about who you should be. And their vision for your life doesn't get to override your actual life.

This chapter is about releasing yourself from the burden of expectations you never agreed to carry.

The Expectation Trap

Expectations are tricky because they're often never explicitly stated. They're just... there. Hovering. Implied. Assumed. And you're supposed to magically know what they are and comply with them without anyone actually having to ask.

Your family expects you to show up for holidays. To visit regularly. To remember birthdays. To participate in family drama. To fulfil whatever role they've cast you in. And if you don't? Well, clearly you don't care about the family.

The problem is: these expectations were never negotiated. You never agreed to them. They were simply imposed and you were expected to comply.

Here's how it works: Someone has an idea about how you should live your life. They never tell you directly. They just assume you know. Then when you fail to meet that unstated expectation, they're disappointed. And somehow, their disappointment becomes your problem.

It's a setup. The expectation was never fair to begin with, but now you're the bad guy for not meeting it.

Examples of unstated family expectations:

- You'll live within 30 minutes of your parents
- You'll have children (and raise them exactly like you were raised)
- You'll pursue a 'respectable' career (translation: one they can brag about)
- You'll be available whenever they need you
- You'll never prioritize your partner/friends over family
- You'll celebrate holidays the way they want to celebrate them
- You'll consult them before making major life decisions
- You'll never change, grow, or become different from who they want you to be

These expectations weren't agreed upon. They were assumed. And now you're supposed to live according to assumptions you never made.

Why Their Disappointment Is Not Your Responsibility

Let me be very clear: disappointing people who have unreasonable expectations is not your fault.

If your parents expected you to live your life according to their blueprint, that's an unreasonable expectation. If they expected you to be available 24/7, that's unreasonable. If they expected you to sacrifice your own dreams for their comfort, that's unreasonable.

And when you fail to meet unreasonable expectations, the resulting disappointment belongs to them. Not you.

You are not responsible for managing their emotional reactions to your very reasonable life choices. You are not required to set yourself on fire to keep them warm. You don't have to shrink your life to fit their expectations.

Here's a radical thought: maybe they should adjust their expectations instead of you adjusting your entire life.

Their disappointment is information about the gap between what they wanted and what reality is. That gap is theirs to reconcile. Not yours to fix by contorting yourself into their fantasy.

You can love someone deeply and still disappoint them. You can care about someone and still choose yourself. You can value the relationship and still refuse to live according to their script.

Their disappointment doesn't mean you're doing something wrong. Sometimes it means you're finally doing something right.

The Scripts They Use

Family members who want to control your life through expectations have a playbook. Let's decode it:

'We just want you to be happy.' Translation: We want you to make choices that make us comfortable, which we've labelled as 'your happiness.'

If they actually wanted you to be happy, they'd support your choices even when those choices differ from their preferences. 'We want you to be happy' followed by criticism of your life choices is not about your happiness. It's about their comfort.

Real support for your happiness looks like: 'I don't understand your choice, but I trust you to know what's best for you.' It doesn't look like: 'I don't understand your choice, so you should change it.'

'Is it too much to ask...' Sometimes, yes. Sometimes what they're asking is way too much. And framing it as a small request doesn't make it one.

'Is it too much to ask you to call every day?' when you have a demanding job, small children, and your own life? Yes, actually, it is. That's a lot. And disguising it as a simple request doesn't change that.

'Is it too much to ask you to spend every holiday with us?' when you have a partner with their own family? Yes. That's asking you to prioritize them over everyone else, always. That's not small.

When someone asks 'Is it too much to ask...', they're trying to make you feel unreasonable for saying no. Don't fall for it. If it feels like too much, it is too much. Your feelings about it are valid.

'We didn't raise you to...' Translation: You're not following the script we wrote for you and we're disappointed.

They didn't raise you to be independent? To make your own choices? To prioritize your own wellbeing? Well, that's on them. You're an adult now. Their raising of you is over. What you do with your life is up to you.

This phrase is designed to make you feel like you're betraying your upbringing by being your own person. You're not. You're just being an adult who makes adult decisions.

'After all we've planned...' Translation: We made plans for your life without asking you, and now we're upset that you're not following them.

Their plans for your life are not binding. They can plan whatever they want. You're not obligated to execute those plans.

Maybe they planned that you'd take over the family business. Maybe they planned where you'd live. Maybe they planned who you'd marry. Those were their plans. Not yours. You don't owe them the fulfilment of plans you never agreed to.

'Don't you care about family?' Translation: Don't you care about family enough to sacrifice your own wellbeing for our preferences?

Caring about family doesn't mean abandoning yourself. It doesn't mean accepting unreasonable demands. It doesn't mean your needs don't matter.

You can care deeply about family while also caring about yourself. Both are possible. Anyone who frames it as either/or is manipulating you.

Setting Your Own Expectations

Here's the radical thing: you get to have your own expectations too. About how you want to be treated. About how much contact feels healthy. About what topics are off-limits. About what role your family plays in your adult life.

Your expectations matter just as much as theirs. Actually, more, because this is your life.

What do you expect from family relationships?

- Mutual respect?
- Support for your choices even when they differ from their preferences?
- Boundaries around certain topics?
- Limited contact?
- Space to live your own life?
- Recognition that you're an autonomous adult?
- Reciprocal effort in maintaining the relationship?

Whatever you expect is valid. And you're allowed to walk away from relationships that don't meet those expectations, even if those relationships are with family.

You're allowed to expect to be treated with respect. You're allowed to expect that your boundaries will be honoured. You're allowed to expect that your choices won't be constantly criticized.

And if family can't meet those very reasonable expectations? That tells you something important about the relationship.

The Consequences of Non-Compliance

When you stop meeting family expectations, there will be consequences. They might pout. Guilt trip. Give you the silent treatment. Talk about you to other family members. Paint you as the problem. Threaten to cut you off (as if that's your loss).

Let them.

You can't control their reactions. You can only control your choices. And if the consequence of living your own life is that your family is upset, that's unfortunate but not catastrophic.

Their disappointment won't kill you. Their disapproval won't kill you. Their silent treatment won't kill you. But abandoning yourself to meet their expectations? That will slowly kill who you are.

So let them have their consequences. Let them be disappointed. Let them adjust their expectations of you. Or not. Either way, you've protected yourself.

Here's what you need to remember: their emotional reactions are theirs to manage. You're not responsible for making them feel better about your choices. You're not obligated to change your life to soothe their disappointment.

They're adults. They can handle disappointment. And if they choose to make that disappointment your problem through manipulation and guilt-tripping, that's information about their emotional maturity, not about whether your choices are valid.

When Expectations Collide

Sometimes, meeting one person's expectations means violating someone else's. Your mother expects you home for Christmas. Your partner's family expects the same. Both can't be met simultaneously.

Or your father expects you to take over the business. Your own dreams lead you somewhere else. One expectation has to be disappointed.

When expectations collide, you have to choose. And here's the hard truth: choose yourself. Choose what aligns with your values, your goals, your wellbeing.

Someone is going to be disappointed no matter what you choose. So you might as well disappoint others while caring for yourself, rather than disappointing yourself while trying to please everyone else.

You cannot meet everyone's expectations. It's literally impossible. And trying to do so will only result in you meeting nobody's expectations. Including your own.

So, make your choices based on what's right for you. Then communicate those choices clearly. Then let other people have their feelings about it.

The Expectation Audit

It's time to get clear on which expectations you're carrying. Try this exercise:

Make a list of all the expectations your family has of you. Everything you 'should' do, be, or want. Write them all down.

Now, next to each one, ask yourself:

• Did I agree to this expectation?

• Does this expectation align with my values and goals?

• Is this expectation reasonable?

• What would happen if I stopped trying to meet this expectation?

• Am I meeting this expectation out of love or out of fear?

The expectations you're meeting out of fear? Those are the ones to examine closely. Fear of disappointing them. Fear of being rejected. Fear of being the bad guy. Fear of conflict.

Those fear-based expectations are probably the ones that need to go. Because you can't build a healthy adult relationship on fear. You can't maintain your own wellbeing while constantly terrified of disappointing others.

The expectations you're meeting out of genuine love and alignment with your values? Keep those. Those aren't burdens. Those are chosen expressions of care.

But the ones you're meeting out of obligation, guilt, or fear? Those are destroying you. And they need to be released.

Communicating Your Non-Compliance

How do you tell your family you're not going to meet their expectations? Ideally: clearly, kindly, and without over-explaining.

Clear: 'I won't be able to do that.' Not 'maybe,' not 'I'll try,' not 'we'll see.' Clear and definitive.

Kind: You don't have to be cruel. You can be firm and kind simultaneously. 'I know this isn't what you hoped for, but this is my decision.'

Brief: Don't JADE (Justify, Argue, Defend, Explain). The more you explain, the more you invite debate. 'This doesn't work for me' is a complete sentence.

Examples:

'I know you expected me to call daily, but I'm not able to do that. I can call weekly on Sundays.'

'I understand you want us to spend every holiday with your family, but we need to split our time. We'll be there for Thanksgiving, but Christmas will be with my partner's family this year.'

'I appreciate that you had plans for me to join the family business, but I'm pursuing a different career. This is my final decision.'

Notice what these have in common: acknowledgment of their expectation, statement of your decision, no apology for the decision, no extensive justification.

You're not asking permission. You're informing them of your choice. There's a difference.

Dealing With the Guilt

You're going to feel guilty. Expect it. Plan for it. Know it's coming.

The guilt doesn't mean you're doing something wrong. It means you're doing something different from what you were programmed to do.

You were programmed to meet their expectations. To make them happy. To prioritize their comfort over your own needs. Violating that programming triggers guilt.

But guilt is just a feeling. It's not a fact. It's not proof that you're wrong. It's just your nervous system's response to breaking old patterns.

Feel the guilt. Acknowledge it. Then do what's right for you anyway.

Over time, the guilt will lessen. As you practice choosing yourself, as you see that the world doesn't end when you disappoint people, as you experience the relief of living according to your own values instead of their expectations. The guilt fades.

It doesn't disappear entirely. But it becomes manageable. It becomes background noise instead of a siren.

The Freedom on the Other Side

Here's what happens when you stop trying to meet everyone's expectations:

You breathe easier. You're not constantly anxious about disappointing someone. You're not carrying the weight of everyone's hopes and dreams for your life.

You make better decisions. When you're not trying to please everyone, you can actually figure out what you want. You can make choices based on your values instead of their preferences.

Your relationships improve. The ones worth keeping, anyway. Because you're showing up authentically instead of performing. You're giving from a place of genuine desire instead of obligation.

You like yourself more. Because you're finally acting in integrity with your own values. Because you're being true to yourself instead of betraying yourself to keep the peace.

You attract better people. People who love you for who you actually are, not for how well you meet their expectations.

This is what's waiting for you on the other side of releasing their expectations. Freedom. Authenticity. Peace.

But you have to be willing to disappoint them to get there. You have to be willing to let their expectations remain unmet. You have to be willing to live your own life even when they wanted you to live theirs.

The Permission You're Waiting For

You don't need their permission to live your own life. You don't need them to agree that your choices are valid. You don't need them to understand why you're not meeting their expectations.

You just need to choose yourself. And then keep choosing yourself, over and over, even when it's uncomfortable.

Their expectations are not your emergency. Their disappointment is not your crisis. Their opinions about your life are just that. Opinions. They don't have to become your reality.

You're allowed to:

- Live where you want
- Pursue the career that fulfils you
- Date/marry who you want (or stay single)
- Have kids or not have kids
- Celebrate holidays how you want
- Set your own priorities
- Make choices they don't understand
- Disappoint them

You're allowed to build a life that makes sense to you, even if it makes no sense to them.

So here's your permission: Stop trying to meet expectations you never agreed to. Stop carrying the weight of their fantasies about who you should be. Stop sacrificing your actual life for their imagined version of your life.

Their expectations are not your emergency. Live accordingly.

Chapter 7: Stop Attending Every Argument You're Invited To

Your family knows exactly which buttons to push because they installed most of them. They know how to bait you. How to provoke you. How to pull you into the same old arguments you've been having for years.

And here's the thing: you don't have to show up.

Just because someone starts an argument doesn't mean you have to participate. Just because they criticize you doesn't mean you have to defend yourself. Just because they want to rehash old conflicts doesn't mean you have to engage.

You are not obligated to attend every argument you're invited to.

This chapter is about recognizing the invitations to fight, declining them gracefully (or not so gracefully), and protecting your peace.

Recognizing the Bait

Family members who want to fight with you don't usually say 'Hey, want to have the same pointless argument we've had 47 times?' They bait you. They make comments. They ask loaded questions. They bring up topics they know will get a rise out of you.

The bait looks like:

• 'So, still single?' (Translation: I'm judging your relationship status)

- 'When are you going to get a real job?' (Translation: I don't respect your career)
- 'Your cousin just bought a house.' (Translation: You're not successful enough)
- 'You're looking tired. Are you taking care of yourself?' (Translation: You look terrible)
- 'I saw an article about [your profession] and it said...' (Translation: Let me tell you what's wrong with your choices)
- 'When I was your age, I already had...' (Translation: You're behind where you should be)
- 'Are you still doing that thing?' (Translation: I hoped you'd have given up by now)

These aren't innocent questions or observations. They're invitations to conflict. They're designed to make you defensive, to pull you into explaining yourself, to engage in the dynamic they want.

Once you learn to recognize bait, you can choose not to take it. You can see it for what it is, manipulation designed to start a fight, and simply decline to participate.

The Anatomy of Family Arguments

Most family arguments follow a predictable pattern. Understanding the pattern helps you interrupt it.

Step 1: The Provocation - Someone makes a comment designed to trigger you. 'When are you going to settle down?'

Step 2: The Reaction - You get defensive. 'My relationship status is none of your business!'

Step 3: The Escalation - 'I'm just concerned about you.' (Escalating while claiming innocence)

Step 4: The Fight - You explain, defend, justify. They double down. It spirals.

Step 5: The Aftermath - Everyone's upset. Nothing is resolved. You'll have this exact fight again in three months.

Here's the thing: you can interrupt this pattern at Step 2. You can choose not to react. You can choose not to defend. You can choose not to engage.

The argument only happens if you participate. And participation is optional.

The Grey Rock Method

When someone is trying to provoke you, give them nothing to work with. Become boring. Uninteresting. As emotionally reactive as a grey rock.

Example:

Them: 'When are you going to get a real job?'

You: 'I'm happy with what I'm doing.'

Them: 'But don't you want to be successful?'

You: 'I'm content with my choices.'

Them: 'I'm just worried about you.'

You: 'I appreciate your concern.'

No defending. No explaining. No justifying. Just bland, neutral responses that don't give them anything to grab onto.

This isn't about being rude. It's about protecting yourself from someone who wants to use your emotional reactions as entertainment or control.

Gray rock works because it removes the payoff. People who start fights do it because they get something out of it. Attention, drama, the satisfaction of getting a rise out of you. When you stop providing that payoff, the behaviour often stops.

Your responses should be:

• Brief (one sentence maximum)

• Neutral (no emotion, no defensiveness)

• Non-engaging (don't ask follow-up questions or offer new topics)

• Repetitive (say the same thing multiple times if needed)

You're not trying to win. You're not trying to convince them. You're just trying to exit the conversation without getting sucked into a fight.

The JADE Mistake

JADE stands for: **Justify, Argue, Defend, Explain**.

And doing any of these things with someone who's not actually interested in understanding you is a waste of your energy.

When you JADE, you're operating from the assumption that if you just explain yourself well enough, they'll understand and respect your choices. But here's the thing: they already understand. They just don't like it.

More explanation won't help. More justification won't work. They're not confused. They're disapproving. And no amount of defending yourself will change that.

Example of JADE-ing:

Them: 'Why aren't you married yet?'

You: 'Well, I've been focused on my career, and I want to make sure I'm with the right person, and marriage isn't a priority for me right now, and I think it's better to wait than to rush into something...'

See what's happening? You're justifying your choices to someone who wasn't asking for information. They were expressing judgment.

Non-JADE response:

Them: 'Why aren't you married yet?'

You: 'I'm not discussing that.'

Done. No explanation. No justification. Just a clear boundary about what you won't discuss.

When you stop JADEing:

- Conversations get shorter
- You waste less energy
- You feel less defensive
- They learn you're not going to engage
- Your boundaries become clearer

Save your explanations for people who actually want to understand you. Everyone else gets a boundary.

Power Dynamics and Family Fights

Most family arguments aren't actually about the stated topic. They're about power. Control. Who gets to decide. Who has to comply. Who's in charge.

Your mother isn't actually concerned about your diet when she comments on your weight. She's trying to assert control. Your father isn't actually worried about your career when he criticizes your choices. He's trying to maintain authority. Your sibling isn't actually interested in your opinion when they start an argument. They're trying to win.

Once you see the power play underneath the argument, it becomes easier to opt out. You're not required to engage in power struggles with people who should be on your side.

The family member who tries to control you through arguments is revealing something important: they believe they have the right to control you. They believe their opinion about your life matters more than your own opinion about your life.

They're wrong. But arguing with them about it won't convince them. The only thing that will convince them is you consistently refusing to engage.

When you stop fighting for your right to make your own choices, you stop implicitly asking for their permission. You're not debating whether you have the right to live your life. You're just living it. Big difference.

Declining the Invitation

So how do you actually opt out of an argument without being rude or causing more conflict?

Scripts for declining arguments:

The Direct Decline: 'I'm not going to discuss this with you.'

Clear. Simple. Not up for negotiation. Works best when you've discussed this boundary before and they're testing it.

The Redirect: 'That's not a conversation I'm having. How about we talk about [different topic]?'

Useful when you want to maintain the interaction but change the subject. Only works if they're willing to let it go.

The Broken Record: 'We clearly see this differently.' (Repeat as needed)

When they keep pushing, just repeat the same neutral statement. Don't elaborate. Don't add new information. Just repeat.

The Acknowledgment Without Agreement: 'I hear that you're upset. I'm still not changing my mind.'

Acknowledges their feelings without engaging with their argument. Useful when they're using emotions to manipulate.

The Topic Boundary: 'This topic isn't up for debate.'

Clear statement that this isn't an open discussion. Works for ongoing issues where they keep trying to relitigate.

The Exit: 'I'm going to go now. We can talk when you're ready to be respectful.'

When they won't stop escalating, you leave. Physically leave the room, end the call, stop responding. This is your nuclear option, but sometimes it's necessary.

After you decline the invitation, stop responding. Don't argue about whether you're going to argue. Don't defend your refusal to engage. Just stop.

They might escalate. They might accuse you of being defensive (ironic, since you're refusing to defend yourself). They might say you're being difficult. Let them. You've declined the invitation. What they do with that is their choice.

When They Won't Let It Go

Some people don't know how to function without conflict. They will keep poking. Keep pushing. Keep trying to pull you into a fight.

Your response: consequences.

'If you continue to bring this up, I'm leaving.'

'If you can't respect my boundary on this topic, we're ending this call.'

'I've told you I'm not discussing this. If you bring it up again, I won't be visiting for a while.'

Then follow through. Every time. Boundaries without enforcement are suggestions. And suggestions get ignored.

The first time you enforce a consequence, they'll be shocked. They're not used to you following through. They're used to you eventually caving.

Don't cave. Hold the line.

Example:

You: 'Mom, I've told you I'm not discussing my relationship. If you bring it up again, I'm ending this call.'

Her: 'But I'm just trying to help. '

You: 'We're done. I'll talk to you next week.' [End call]

No second chances in the moment. No warnings after you've already warned them. Just immediate follow-through.

This feels harsh. It feels mean. It feels like you're overreacting.

You're not. You stated a clear boundary. They violated it. You enforced the consequence. That's not mean. That's healthy.

The Silent Treatment (And How to Not Fall For It)

Some family members will punish your refusal to argue by giving you the silent treatment. They'll withdraw, ignore you, freeze you out.

This is emotional abuse designed to make you so uncomfortable that you'll abandon your boundary to make it stop.

Don't.

The silent treatment is a manipulation tactic. It's punishment for not complying. It's designed to train you to fear their withdrawal so you'll do whatever they want to avoid it.

Your response to the silent treatment:

- Nothing.

That's it. Just let them have their tantrum. Use the silence to rest. Enjoy the peace. Don't chase them. Don't apologize for your boundary. Don't try to fix it.

They'll come back when they realize it's not working. When they realize you're not suffering without their attention. When they figure out that silent treatment doesn't make you cave.

And when they come back, don't pretend nothing happened. 'I'm glad you're ready to talk again. My boundary about [topic] still stands.'

Don't reward the silent treatment by acting like everything's fine. Acknowledge what happened. Restate your boundary. Move forward.

The Boundary Testing

After you've set a boundary about not arguing certain topics, family will test it. They'll 'forget.' They'll claim they 'didn't know.' They'll bring it up 'accidentally.'

They're not forgetting. They're testing to see if you'll enforce the boundary.

Enforce it immediately:

'As I mentioned, I don't discuss that topic. Let's talk about something else or I'm going to end this call.'

Then follow through if they continue. Every single time.

Consistency is everything. If you enforce the boundary Monday but let it slide Friday, you've taught them that the boundary is negotiable. That if they push enough, you'll cave.

Don't negotiate. Don't make exceptions. Don't let things slide 'just this once.' Hold the line every single time.

When Arguments Serve a Purpose

For some families, arguing is connection. It's how they interact. It's how they feel close. Dysfunction is their normal.

When you refuse to argue, they might feel rejected. Like you don't want to engage with them. Like you're pulling away from the family.

That's unfortunate. But it's not your problem to fix.

You're not obligated to participate in dysfunctional connection just because that's what they're used to. You're allowed to want healthy connection. You're allowed to refuse the old pattern.

They can learn to connect with you in healthier ways. Or they can't. Either way, you're not required to engage in dysfunction to maintain the relationship.

If the only way they know how to connect is through conflict, that's something they need to work on. Not something you need to accommodate.

Different Types of Arguments to Avoid

Not all arguments are created equal. Some are worth having. Most aren't. Here are the types to avoid:

The Re-litigator: Arguments about things that happened years ago that can't be changed. 'Remember when you...'

Response: 'I'm not relitigating the past. What's done is done.'

The Opinion Police: Arguments about your personal choices that don't affect them. Your career, your relationship, your body, your beliefs.

Response: 'I'm not debating my personal choices.'

The Hypothetical: Arguments about things that might happen in the future. 'What if you...'

Response: 'I'm not arguing about hypotheticals.'

The Unwinnable: Arguments where they're not actually interested in your perspective. They just want to convince you they're right.

Response: 'We see this differently. I'm okay with that.'

The Bait and Switch: They start with one topic then pivot to what they really want to fight about.

Response: 'This conversation has shifted to a topic I'm not discussing. We're done.'

The Performance: Arguments that happen in front of others to recruit allies or make you look bad.

Response: 'This isn't the time or place. We can discuss this privately later if you want.'

The Peaceful Option

Refusing to argue doesn't mean you don't care. It doesn't mean you're avoiding conflict. It means you've learned that some arguments are designed to go nowhere, serve no purpose, and only damage the relationship.

You can love someone and refuse to fight with them. You can care about someone and decline to defend yourself to them. You can maintain a relationship while opting out of destructive patterns.

Not every argument deserves your participation. Not every criticism requires a response. Not every provocation needs to be met with defence.

You have better things to do with your energy than re-enact the same pointless conflicts over and over. Your peace is more important than winning. Your wellbeing is more important than being right.

So stop attending arguments you're invited to. Decline politely. Or decline impolitely. Either way, decline.

Your presence at every family argument is not required. Really. It's optional.

The Long-Term Benefit

Here's what happens when you consistently refuse to argue:

They stop trying. Eventually. Once they realize that you won't engage, that you won't defend, that you won't participate, they stop inviting you to fight. It's not fun anymore when you won't play.

The relationship might actually improve. Without the constant conflict, there's space for actual connection. For conversations that don't end in fights. For interactions that leave you feeling good instead of drained.

Or the relationship might end. If fighting was the only way they knew how to connect with you, and you refuse to fight, they might not know what to do with you. That's sad. But it's also information.

Either way, you've protected your peace. You've refused to participate in dysfunction. You've chosen yourself.

And that's worth more than winning any argument.

PART THREE

FRIENDS & SOCIAL DYNAMICS

Chapter 8: You are Attracting Your Family Dynamic in Your Friendships

Here's the uncomfortable truth: you're recreating your family dynamics in your friendships. The patterns you learned at home, the ones you swore you'd never repeat, are showing up in how you choose friends, what you tolerate, and what role you play.

That friend who takes and never gives? They're your self-absorbed parent. That friend who criticizes everything you do? They're your critical parent. That friend who needs constant emotional support but disappears when you need them? They're your parentified child dynamic all over again.

You're not doing this consciously. Your nervous system is doing it. It's seeking what's familiar. And unfortunately, if your family was dysfunctional, dysfunction feels like home.

This chapter is about recognizing the patterns, understanding why you keep attracting the same dynamics, and learning to choose differently.

The Roles You Keep Playing

In your family, you had a role. The good child. The scapegoat. The peacekeeper. The parentified child. The lost child. And unless you've consciously worked to change it, you're still playing that role in your friendships.

The Caretaker: You're always the one giving support, solving problems, managing crises. Your friends call when they need something but are mysteriously unavailable when you do.

This is the parentified child grown up. You learned that your value comes from being useful, so you unconsciously seek out friends who need saving. Friends who have constant drama. Friends who are always in crisis. Friends who take and take and take.

And you give because that's what you know. Because caretaking feels like love. Because being needed feels like being valued.

But here's the thing: you're exhausted. You're resentful. And somewhere deep down, you know this isn't real friendship. It's you performing the same role you learned in childhood.

The Comedian: You're the funny one. The entertaining one. The one who makes everyone laugh. But nobody knows the real you because you're always performing.

This is often the lost child or the family scapegoat's adaptation. You learned that being entertaining kept you safe. That humour deflected from pain. That making others happy was your job.

So now you have friends who love your humour but don't actually know you. Who enjoy your company but wouldn't notice if you were struggling. Who appreciate the show but don't see the person.

The Peacekeeper: You smooth over conflicts, mediate disagreements, make sure everyone gets along. You're stressed anytime there's tension in the group.

This is the family mediator pattern. You learned that conflict is dangerous and that your job is to keep everyone happy. So you unconsciously gravitate toward friend groups with drama, where you can play your familiar role.

You're not maintaining peace. You're managing everyone's emotions while ignoring your own. Again.

The Accommodator: You're always flexible. Always available. Always willing to change your plans. You never say no, never express preferences, never cause inconvenience.

This is the good child pattern. You learned that your needs don't matter as much as everyone else's. That being low-maintenance is valuable. That having preferences makes you difficult.

So you have friendships where you always adjust. Where you go along with whatever everyone else wants. Where your opinion is never sought because everyone knows you'll just agree anyway.

The Friends You Keep Choosing

You're not randomly selecting friends. You're unconsciously attracted to people who recreate your family dynamic. Because that's what feels normal. That's what your nervous system recognizes as 'connection.'

The Taker: This friend calls when they need something. Advice, support, a favour, an audience for their drama. But when you need them? They're busy. They're dealing with their own stuff. They'll get back to you (they won't).

If you had a self-absorbed parent, takers feel familiar. You're used to relationships being one-way streets. You're used to giving without receiving. You're used to your needs coming last.

So when a friend takes and takes, it doesn't immediately register as wrong. It just feels like relationship. Like this is how it works. Like this is your role.

The Critic: This friend is always pointing out what you're doing wrong, how you could be better, what you should change. They frame it as 'being honest' or 'helping you grow,' but it feels like constant judgment.

If you had a critical parent, critics feel like intimacy. You're used to criticism being packaged as care. You're used to feeling like you're never quite good enough. You're used to working for approval you'll never fully receive.

So when a friend criticizes you constantly, you don't set a boundary. You just try harder. You work to prove yourself. You accept that this is what friendship looks like.

The Drama Magnet: This friend always has a crisis. Always needs rescuing. Always has chaos swirling around them. And somehow, it becomes your job to fix it.

If you were parentified as a child, drama magnets feel like purpose. You're used to being the fixer. The problem-solver. The one who handles everything. You're uncomfortable when things are calm because you don't know who to be without a crisis to manage.

So you unconsciously seek out friends with constant drama. Because that's where you feel useful. That's where you know your role. That's where you feel needed.

The Inconsistent One: This friend is hot and cold. Close one day, distant the next. Makes plans then cancels. Says they care but their actions don't match.

If you had an inconsistent or unpredictable parent, this feels like love. You're used to working for attention. You're used to not knowing where you stand. You're used to earning affection instead of receiving it freely.

So when a friend is inconsistent, you don't walk away. You just try harder. You work to be valuable enough that they'll stick around. You accept breadcrumbs and call it friendship.

Why Healthy Friendships Feel Wrong

Here's the really messed up part: when you encounter a healthy friendship, one where both people give and receive, where there's mutual respect, where your needs matter as much as theirs, it feels weird. Uncomfortable. Suspicious.

You don't trust it. You wait for the other shoe to drop. You wonder what they want. You feel like you need to earn their care.

Because healthy doesn't feel like home. Dysfunction feels like home. So your nervous system keeps pulling you back toward what's familiar, even when what's familiar is harmful.

Signs a friendship is healthy (and why they might feel wrong):

- They remember what you tell them about your life (feels like: 'Why are they paying such close attention?')
- They check in on you without needing something (feels like: 'What do they want from me?')
- They respect your boundaries without making you feel guilty (feels like: 'This is too easy, something's wrong')

• They celebrate your wins without making it about them (feels like: 'Why aren't they jealous or competitive?')

• They apologize when they hurt you (feels like: 'Is this a trap?')

• They're consistent and reliable (feels like: 'This can't last')

If healthy friendship feels foreign, that's information about what you learned was normal. It's not information about what's actually healthy.

The Friendship Audit

It's time to look at your friendships honestly. Not to judge yourself, but to see the patterns clearly.

For each significant friendship, ask yourself:

• Do I feel energized or drained after spending time with this person?

• Is this friendship reciprocal, or am I doing most of the work?

• Can I be authentic with this person, or am I performing?

• Do they support my growth, or do they keep me small?

• Do they respect my boundaries, or do they push against them?

• What role am I playing in this friendship?

• Does this dynamic remind me of any family relationship?

Be honest. Really honest. Not 'but they mean well' honest. Not 'they're going through a hard time' honest. Actually honest.

If you're constantly exhausted by a friendship, that's data. If you feel like you can't be yourself, that's data. If it's always one-sided, that's data. If it feels like work instead of connection, that's data.

Use it.

Breaking the Pattern

Understanding the pattern is step one. Changing it is step two. Here's how:

1. Recognize your role: Name it. 'I'm playing the caretaker again.' 'I'm being the accommodator.' 'I'm seeking approval like I did from my critical parent.' Awareness interrupts automatic behaviour.

2. Notice what feels familiar: When you meet someone new, pay attention to whether they feel immediately comfortable or slightly unfamiliar. If they feel like instant best friends, ask yourself: 'Do they feel familiar because they're actually healthy, or because they're triggering my old patterns?'

3. Choose differently: Consciously seek out people who don't fit your old patterns. People who are healthy in ways that make you uncomfortable. People who offer reciprocity. People who respect boundaries. Even if it feels weird.

4. Practice reciprocal friendship: Start asking for support. Start expressing needs. Start expecting that friendship goes both ways. It will feel uncomfortable. Do it anyway.

5. Set boundaries in existing friendships: With friends who are taking too much, start saying no. With friends who are critical, start calling it out. With friends who are inconsistent, start expecting more. Some will adjust. Some won't.

6. Let go of what's not working: Some friendships can't be salvaged because they were built on a dysfunctional dynamic. If the only way to maintain the friendship is to keep playing your old role, it might be time to let it go.

What Healthy Friendship Actually Looks Like

Healthy friendship is:

• Reciprocal: Both people give and receive. Both people initiate. Both people show up.

• Respectful: Boundaries are honoured. Differences are accepted. Privacy is maintained.

• Supportive: You celebrate each other's wins without jealousy. You comfort each other's losses without making it about you.

• Authentic: You can be real with each other. You don't have to perform or pretend.

• Balanced: Neither person is always the giver or always the taker. The relationship feels equitable over time.

• Consistent: They show up. They follow through. They're reliable.

• Growth-oriented: They encourage your growth, even when it means you're changing.

If this sounds foreign, start small. You don't have to overhaul all your friendships overnight. Just start noticing the patterns. Start choosing one thing differently. Start expecting a little more reciprocity.

The Grief of Seeing Clearly

Once you start seeing these patterns, you can't unsee them. And that's painful. Because it means recognizing that some of your friendships aren't actually healthy. That some of your closest friends are recreating your family dysfunction. That you've been accepting crumbs and calling it connection.

Grieve that. It's a real loss. The loss of illusion. The loss of relationships you thought were solid. The loss of the comfort of familiar patterns, even when those patterns were harmful.

But on the other side of that grief is clarity. Is the possibility of actual healthy friendships. Is the freedom to choose differently.

You're not doomed to repeat your family patterns in your friendships. But you do have to become conscious of them. You do have to be willing to see them clearly. You do have to be brave enough to choose differently, even when different feels uncomfortable.

Your friendships can be different from your family. But first, you have to stop unconsciously recreating your family in your friendships.

Chapter 9: Stop Letting People Insult You in the Name of Friendship

'I'm just being honest.' 'I'm just joking.' 'Don't be so sensitive.' 'That's just how I am.' 'You know I love you, but...'

These are the phrases people use when they want to insult you without consequences. When they want to be cruel without being held accountable. When they want to violate your boundaries while pretending to be a good friend.

And if you've been socialized to be nice, to be accommodating, to not make waves, you probably let it slide. You laugh it off. You tell yourself they didn't mean it. You make excuses for behaviour you would never tolerate from a stranger.

Stop.

Real friends don't disguise insults as honesty. Real friends don't use humour as a weapon. Real friends don't make you feel small and then tell you you're too sensitive.

This chapter is about recognizing when 'friendship' is just abuse with a social excuse, and learning to protect yourself from people who hide behind the label of 'friend' while treating you terribly.

The Disguised Insult Playbook

Let's decode the ways people insult you while pretending to be your friend:

'I'm just being honest.' Translation: I'm about to say something mean and I want you to thank me for it.

Honesty doesn't require cruelty. You can tell someone the truth without being insulting. When someone prefaces a statement with 'I'm just being honest,' they're usually about to say something unnecessarily harsh and they want credit for their 'honesty' instead of consequences for their cruelty.

Real honesty sounds like: 'I'm concerned about this thing I've noticed. Can we talk about it?' Fake honesty sounds like: 'Well, honestly, you've really let yourself go.'

One is care. The other is criticism disguised as care.

'I'm just joking.' Translation: I just insulted you and I want you to pretend it didn't hurt.

Jokes are supposed to be funny. If you're the only one not laughing, it's not a joke. It's mockery. And when someone says 'I'm just joking' after saying something hurtful, they're trying to make your hurt your problem instead of their cruelty their responsibility.

Real jokes don't consistently target the same person. Real jokes don't hit on your deepest insecurities. Real jokes don't require you to develop a thick skin to tolerate your friends.

If someone's 'jokes' always come at your expense, they're not joking. They're insulting you and expecting you to smile about it.

'Don't be so sensitive.' Translation: I want to say whatever I want without considering your feelings, and I'm going to blame you for having feelings about it.

When someone tells you not to be so sensitive after they've hurt you, they're refusing to take responsibility for their impact. They're making your legitimate reaction to their poor behaviour into your problem.

You're not too sensitive. They're not being sensitive enough to the impact of their words. Big difference.

'That's just how I am.' Translation: I'm not going to change my hurtful behaviour, so you need to just accept it.

'That's just how I am' is not a free pass to treat people poorly. It's not an excuse. It's not a valid defence. It's a refusal to grow or take accountability.

Your response: 'And this is just how I am. Someone who doesn't tolerate being insulted.'

'You know I love you, but...' Translation: I'm about to say something hurtful and I want the word 'love' to negate the damage.

Love doesn't excuse cruelty. Saying 'I love you' before or after an insult doesn't make it not an insult. It's just manipulation designed to make you feel like you can't call out the behaviour without rejecting their 'love.'

Real love doesn't require a 'but.' Real love doesn't come with constant criticism. Real love doesn't feel like death by a thousand cuts.

The 'Brutal Honesty' Con

Some people wear their 'brutal honesty' like a badge of honour. They pride themselves on 'telling it like it is.'

They think being unfiltered is a personality trait to celebrate.

It's not. It's just rudeness with PR.

Being brutally honest usually just means being brutal. Because honest doesn't require harsh. You can be truthful without being cruel. You can give feedback without being insulting. You can disagree without being disrespectful.

People who pride themselves on brutal honesty are usually just people who enjoy being brutal and hide behind 'honesty' to avoid accountability.

Notice who they're 'brutally honest' with. Is it everyone? Or is it specifically people who are socialized to accept poor treatment? People who won't fight back? People who can be relied upon to absorb the cruelty without consequences?

Brutally honest people are rarely brutally honest with their boss. Or with people who will call them out. They save their 'honesty' for people they know will tolerate it.

That's not honesty. That's targeting.

The Joke That's Not a Joke

Let's talk about the friend who constantly makes jokes at your expense. About your weight, your job, your relationship status, your choices, your appearance. And when you say it hurts, they tell you to lighten up.

That's not a friend. That's a bully with a laugh track.

Real friendly teasing:

- Is reciprocal (everyone gets teased equally)
- Avoids deep insecurities
- Stops when someone says they're uncomfortable
- Comes from a place of affection, not malice
- Is actually funny to everyone, including the target

Bullying disguised as joking:

- Consistently targets the same person
- Hits on known insecurities and vulnerabilities
- Continues even when the target isn't laughing
- Has an edge of meanness, not playfulness
- Makes the target feel small, not included

If you dread seeing this friend because you know they're going to 'joke' about something you're sensitive about, that's not friendship. That's abuse with an audience.

Why You're Tolerating This

You're tolerating insults disguised as friendship because you've been trained to tolerate poor treatment in the name of keeping the peace, not being difficult, and maintaining relationships.

You've been told:

- Don't be so sensitive
- Learn to take a joke
- They're just trying to help
- They mean well
- That's just their sense of humour

• You're overreacting

All of these messages teach you that the problem is your reaction, not their action. That you should adjust your feelings, not that they should adjust their behaviour.

But here's the truth: you're not too sensitive. You're having a normal reaction to being treated poorly. And the fact that it's packaged as 'honesty' or 'humour' or 'friendship' doesn't make it acceptable.

You've also been taught that friendships are scarce and valuable and should be maintained at all costs. That losing a friend is a failure. That you should work to keep people in your life even when they're hurting you.

That's wrong. Some friendships should end. Some people should be removed from your life. And tolerating abuse to maintain a friendship is not loyalty. It's self-betrayal.

Setting Boundaries With 'Honest' Friends

When someone insults you and disguises it as honesty, friendship, or humour, you have options:

Call it out directly: 'That was hurtful.' 'That wasn't funny.' 'I don't appreciate being spoken to that way.'

Don't soften it. Don't apologize for having feelings. Don't make it easier for them by downplaying your hurt. Just state the fact: that hurt.

Refuse the excuse: When they say 'I'm just being honest' or 'I'm just joking,' respond with: 'You're being cruel.' 'You're being disrespectful.' 'Honesty doesn't require insults.'

Don't accept their reframing. Name what's actually happening.

Set a clear boundary: 'Don't comment on my weight.' 'Don't make jokes about my relationship status.' 'Don't criticize my career choices.' 'If you continue to speak to me this way, I'm leaving.'

Specific boundaries about specific behaviours. Then enforce them.

Leave the conversation: If they continue after you've set a boundary, leave. End the call. Walk away. Stop responding to texts.

You told them the behaviour wasn't acceptable. They chose to continue. You're not obligated to keep subjecting yourself to it.

How They'll Respond

When you stop accepting insults disguised as friendship, the insulter will likely:

Double down: 'See, I knew you couldn't handle the truth.' 'You're being ridiculous.' 'I can't believe you're making such a big deal out of nothing.'

This is manipulation designed to make you question your reality. Don't. You know what you heard. You know how it made you feel. Trust that.

Play victim: 'I guess I'm just a terrible friend.' 'Fine, I won't ever be honest with you again.' 'I was just trying to help.'

This is designed to make you comfort them for hurting you. Don't. Let them have their feelings. Your boundary stands.

Recruit others: 'Can you believe how sensitive they're being?' 'I was just being honest and they freaked out.'

They'll try to get mutual friends to side with them. Some will. That tells you who else you need to create distance from.

Temporarily improve: They'll be nice for a while. Careful. Thoughtful. Then slowly the behaviour will creep back in, testing if you'll still enforce the boundary.

Enforce it again. Every time. Consistency is everything.

When the Whole Friend Group Is Toxic

Sometimes it's not just one friend. It's the whole dynamic. The group bonding is based on mockery, on roasting each other, on seeing who can take the most abuse without flinching.

And if you can't take it, you're told you don't fit. You're too sensitive for the group. You can't hang.

Here's the thing: maybe you can't hang with this group. Maybe you shouldn't. Maybe this group's idea of friendship is toxic and you're finally seeing it clearly.

Healthy friend groups don't require you to have thick skin. They don't bond over cruelty. They don't make you feel like you have to prove you can tolerate abuse to belong.

If the whole group dynamic is built on insults, mockery, and meanness, you're not losing good friends by leaving. You're escaping a toxic environment.

The Difference Between Honesty and Cruelty

Because someone will say: 'But how do I know if my friend is being cruel or genuinely trying to help?'

Here's how:

Genuine honesty:

- Is offered with kindness
- Comes from a place of care, not judgment
- Is about specific behaviour, not your entire character
- Offers support or solutions, not just criticism
- Respects your autonomy to make your own choices
- Stops when you say you've heard enough

Cruelty disguised as honesty:

- Has an edge of meanness or superiority
- Feels more like judgment than care
- Attacks your character, not specific actions
- Offers only criticism, no support
- Assumes they know better than you about your own life
- Continues even when you've asked them to stop

One feels like support, even when it's hard to hear. The other feels like attack.

Trust your gut. You know the difference.

When to Walk Away

Not everyone will respect your boundaries about how you want to be treated. Some people are committed to their right to insult you more than they're committed to the friendship.

Signs this friendship needs to end:

• They refuse to stop insulting you even after you've clearly asked them to

• They mock you for having boundaries

• They recruit others to gang up on you

• The 'jokes' get meaner after you ask them to stop

• They gaslight you about what was said or how it was meant

• You dread spending time with them

• You feel worse about yourself after every interaction

• The entire relationship is built on them criticizing you

If most of those are true, this isn't a friendship worth saving. It's a toxic relationship you're holding onto out of habit, history, or fear of being alone.

Let it go.

What Real Friendship Feels Like

Real friends can give you honest feedback without making you feel like garbage. Real friends can joke with you without targeting your insecurities. Real friends make you feel better about yourself, not worse.

Real friendship:

- Builds you up more than it tears you down
- Feels safe, not like you're walking on eggshells
- Involves kindness, not constant criticism
- Respects your boundaries without making it a big deal
- Allows you to be yourself without fear of mockery

If you don't have friendships like that right now, it's not because they don't exist. It's because you've been tolerating friendships that fall far short of that standard.

Raise your standards. Stop accepting insults in the name of friendship. Stop making excuses for people who consistently make you feel bad.

You deserve friends who are actually kind to you. Not friends who hide their cruelty behind 'honesty' or 'humour.' Actual kind friends.

But you won't find them until you stop tolerating the ones who aren't.

Chapter 10: You Don't Have to Eat That Cake

Someone baked a cake. Or brought cookies. Or ordered pizza for the group. Or planned an activity you don't want to do. Or scheduled a get-together you don't want to attend.

And now there's pressure. Subtle or not-so-subtle pressure to participate, to join in, to be a good sport, to not be difficult.

'Come on, just one piece.' 'Don't be boring.' 'You have to try it, I made it special for you.' 'Everyone else is doing it.' 'You're no fun anymore.'

Here's what you need to know: You don't have to eat the cake.

This chapter is about resisting social pressure to do things you don't want to do, even when everyone else thinks you should, even when it seems like a small thing, even when refusing feels awkward.

The Social Pressure to Comply

Social groups have norms. Expectations. Unspoken rules about what makes you a good member of the group. And one of those rules is usually: go along to get along.

Don't be difficult. Don't make it weird. Don't be the one who can't just relax and have fun. Don't be high maintenance. Don't make people accommodate you. Just participate.

So you eat food you don't want because someone will be offended if you don't. You stay at events longer than you want because leaving early makes you the bad guy. You participate in activities you don't enjoy because opting out means you're not a team player.

You prioritize everyone else's comfort over your own preferences. Over and over. Until you're not even sure what your preferences are anymore because you're so used to ignoring them.

Why This Matters (It's Not Really About Cake)

This isn't actually about cake. It's about your right to say no to things you don't want, even when those things seem small or trivial.

Because if you can't say no to cake, how are you going to say no to:

- A job offer that's wrong for you but makes your family proud
- A relationship that's comfortable but unfulfilling
- Living in a place you hate because your friends are there
- Attending events that drain you because you 'should'
- Participating in group activities you genuinely don't enjoy

The cake is practice. It's the lowest stakes version of 'can you honour your own preferences even when there's social pressure not to?'

And if you can't do it with cake, you probably can't do it with bigger things either.

The Scripts They Use

Let's decode the social pressure tactics:

'Just try it.' Translation: Your no doesn't count. I'm going to keep pushing until you give in.

'Just try it' sounds reasonable. It sounds like they're not asking for much. But you already said no. They heard you. They're just hoping that if they push a little more, you'll cave.

Don't. 'No thank you' is a complete sentence. You don't owe anyone a taste.

'I made it special for you.' Translation: I'm going to guilt you into compliance by making my effort your obligation.

Maybe they did make it for you. Or maybe they're just saying that to create obligation. Either way, you didn't ask them to. Their effort doesn't create your obligation to consume it.

'That was thoughtful, but I'm not eating cake right now. Thank you though.'

'Don't be boring/no fun/difficult.' Translation: Conform to group behaviour or be labelled as the problem.

This is social ostracism as a compliance tool. The threat is: if you don't participate, you'll be seen as not fun, and maybe you won't be included next time.

Maybe you won't be. If a group only includes people who always say yes to everything, that's not a group you want to be part of anyway.

'Everyone else is doing it.' Translation: Peer pressure.

Cool. Everyone else can do what they want. That doesn't obligate you to join.

You're not everyone else. You're you. And you get to make different choices.

'It's rude to refuse.' Translation: Your preferences are less important than social conventions.

What's actually rude is continuing to push after someone has said no. What's actually rude is prioritizing your desire for compliance over their clearly stated preference.

Declining politely is not rude. Pushing someone after they've declined is.

Your Right to Say No

You are allowed to:

- Decline food for any reason or no reason
- Leave events early (or not attend at all)
- Opt out of group activities
- Have different preferences than everyone else
- Not explain or justify your choices
- Disappoint people who expected your compliance

You don't need a good reason. You don't need any reason. 'I don't want to' is sufficient.

You're not obligated to eat, drink, participate, stay, or engage just because someone else wants you to. Even if they're your friend. Even if they put in effort. Even if everyone else is doing it.

Your body, your time, your choices. Always.

How to Say No Without Apologizing

Here's the thing: you've probably been taught to soften your no. To apologize for it. To explain it. To make it easier for the other person to accept.

Stop.

A clear, polite no doesn't require apology or explanation:

- 'No thank you.'
- 'I'm good, thanks.'
- 'Not for me, but you enjoy!'
- 'I'm going to pass.'
- 'I'm heading out now. See you next time!'

Notice what these don't include: apologies, explanations, justifications, or invitations for them to convince you otherwise.

If they push:

- 'I appreciate the offer, but no.'
- 'I'm not eating that, but thank you.'
- 'No' works for me.'

Still no explanation. Still no apology. Just a repeated, clear boundary.

And if they keep pushing after that? They're being rude, not you. At that point, you can just stop responding. You've said no. You don't have to keep defending it.

The JADE Trap (Again)

When you explain why you're saying no, you invite debate. You give them ammunition to argue with your reason.

'I'm not eating cake because I'm trying to eat healthier.'

'Oh come on, one piece won't hurt! You're already so healthy! Live a little!'

See? Your reason became something to argue with.

But if you just say 'No thank you' with no reason given, there's nothing to argue with. Your no is your no. Not up for debate.

Don't JADE (Justify, Argue, Defend, Explain). Just decline and move on.

When the Group Makes It Weird

Sometimes when you opt out, the group makes it A Thing. They comment on it. They make a big deal about your choice. They make you feel like you're ruining the vibe just by having a preference.

'Oh, you're not drinking? Why? Are you okay? What's wrong? Come on, just one drink!'

Your choice becomes the centre of attention. And now everyone's looking at you. And you feel like you have to justify yourself or give in to make it stop.

Don't. Hold your boundary and let it be weird.

'I'm not drinking tonight. How about that weather?' [Change subject]

Or even more directly: 'I'm not discussing my reasons. Anyone want to talk about [different topic]?'

The awkwardness they're creating is theirs to manage, not yours to fix by giving in. You stated your preference. They're the ones making it weird by not accepting it.

Let them be uncomfortable with your boundary. That's not your problem to solve.

The Food-Specific Dynamics

Food is particularly fraught with social pressure because sharing food is culturally coded as connection, love, and community. Refusing food can feel like refusing the relationship.

But it's not. You can connect without eating. You can appreciate someone's effort without consuming what they made. You can participate in the gathering without eating everything offered.

Special considerations with food:

Dietary restrictions: You don't have to explain your dietary choices. 'This doesn't work for me' is enough. You don't owe anyone details about your health, allergies, or preferences.

Diet culture pressure: Comments about your food choices are inappropriate. 'Should you be eating that?' or 'You're so good for not having any!' are both judgmental and unwelcome. Shut it down: 'Please don't comment on what I eat.'

Cultural food expectations: Some cultures show love through food, and refusing can feel like rejecting that love. You can appreciate the gesture without consuming the food: 'This looks beautiful, thank you for thinking of me. I'm not eating right now but I appreciate the care.'

When It Is Not Just Cake

The same dynamics apply to any social expectation:

Events: You don't have to attend everything. You don't have to stay for the whole thing. You can arrive late or leave early or not go at all.

'I can't make it, but have fun!' No explanation needed.

Activities: You don't have to participate in group activities you don't enjoy. You can opt out of the team building exercise, the group hike, the karaoke night.

'That's not my thing, but you all have fun!' Then do something else or go home.

Gifts: You don't have to pretend to love a gift you don't like. You can be gracious without lying.

'Thank you for thinking of me!' is true even if you hate the actual gift.

Plans: You don't have to agree to plans you don't want to do just because everyone else wants to.

'That doesn't work for me. You all go ahead!' Then make different plans or enjoy your solo time.

The Boundary Holders

When you start saying no to things everyone expects you to say yes to, you'll find out who in your group respects boundaries and who doesn't.

Boundary respecters:

- Accept your no without pushing
- Don't make a big deal about your different choice
- Don't take your no personally
- Continue to include you even when you opt out sometimes

Boundary violators:

- Push back on your no
- Make your choice about them
- Guilt trip or pressure you to comply
- Withdraw or punish when you don't participate

This information is valuable. It tells you who's safe to have boundaries with and who isn't. It tells you who sees you as an autonomous person and who sees you as someone who should always comply.

Keep the boundary respecters close. Create distance from the boundary violators.

The Long-Term Benefits

What happens when you start honouring your own preferences, even in small things like cake?

You learn that saying no doesn't kill you. That disappointing people is survivable. That the world doesn't end when you have a different preference than everyone else.

You build the muscle of self-respect. Of treating your own wants and needs as legitimate. Of not automatically sacrificing your preferences for social harmony.

You attract better people. People who respect boundaries. People who don't need you to always say yes. People who value your authenticity more than your compliance.

You become more yourself. Less of a people-pleaser. Less concerned with what everyone thinks. More connected to what you actually want.

All from saying no to cake.

Not because the cake matters. But because your right to say no matters. Your right to have preferences matters. Your right to disappoint people matters.

So start small. Start with cake. Or with leaving an event early. Or with opting out of one activity.

Practice saying no. Practice not explaining. Practice tolerating the mild social awkwardness of having a boundary.

Because if you can't say no to cake, you can't say no to anything.

And you deserve to be able to say no.

Chapter 11: It is Okay If They Don't Like You

Not everyone is going to like you. Not everyone is going to approve of you. Not everyone is going to think you're great. And that's not just okay. It's inevitable.

But if you're someone who was raised to believe that being liked was your primary job, this is terrifying. If you learned that your worth depended on approval, the idea of someone not liking you feels like death.

It's not. It's just information. Information that not everyone is your person. Not everyone will get you. Not everyone needs to.

This chapter is about releasing yourself from the exhausting burden of trying to be universally liked and learning to be okay with disapproval.

The Approval Trap

If you're reading this, you probably care a lot about being liked. You probably spend significant energy trying to make sure people approve of you. You probably adjust yourself, your opinions, your personality, your choices, based on your audience.

You learned this young. You learned that love was conditional on good behaviour, on achievement, on being pleasant, on not causing problems. You learned that approval was something you earned, not something you received freely.

So now you're an adult who:

• Struggles to express opinions that might be unpopular

- Changes your personality based on who you're with
- Overthinks every social interaction
- Feels crushed when someone doesn't like you
- Can't handle criticism without spiralling
- Makes yourself smaller to make others comfortable
- Avoids conflict at all costs
- Needs constant reassurance that you're okay/good/liked

This is exhausting. And it's impossible. Because you cannot be everything to everyone. You cannot make everyone like you. You cannot earn universal approval.

And trying to do so means you're living a half-life, constantly performing, never fully yourself.

Why Universal Approval Is Impossible

Even if you could perfectly mould yourself to what each person wants, you still wouldn't be universally liked. Because:

People have conflicting preferences: What one person loves about you, another will hate. You can't be both loud and quiet, both assertive and accommodating, both ambitious and relaxed. Different people want different things.

Some people project onto you: Sometimes people don't like you because you remind them of someone else, or because they're insecure about something you represent, or because they're having a bad day and you're there. It's not about you.

Your values will conflict with others: If you have strong values, some people will disagree with those values. And that's fine. You're not looking for universal agreement. You're looking for alignment with people who share your values.

Some people just won't vibe with you: And that's okay. Not everyone has to. Chemistry is a thing. Compatibility is a thing. Sometimes there's just no connection, and nobody's wrong. You're just not each other's people.

Trying to be liked by everyone is trying to be bland enough to offend no one. And that means being interesting to no one. Including yourself.

The Cost of People-Pleasing

What are you sacrificing to try to be universally liked?

- Your authentic opinions and beliefs
- Your personality and quirks
- Your boundaries and preferences
- Your time and energy
- Your self-respect
- Your ability to connect deeply with anyone

People-pleasing creates surface-level connections with everyone and deep connections with no one. Because people can't connect with a mask. They can only connect with the real you.

And if you're always performing, always adjusting, always trying to be what they want, they're not connecting with you. They're connecting with your performance. And you're alone even when you're with people.

That's the real cost. Not that people won't like you. But that even when they do, it doesn't matter, because they don't actually know you.

What Happens When You Stop Trying

When you stop trying to be liked by everyone, something magical happens: you start being actually liked by some people. Deeply liked. Really known and appreciated.

Because when you show up authentically, quirks, opinions, boundaries, and all, you repel people who aren't your people. And you attract people who are.

The people who don't like the real you were never going to be genuine connections anyway. You were just performing for them. Losing their approval isn't actually losing anything real.

But the people who like the real you? Those connections are real. Those relationships are sustainable. Those people are actually seeing you, not the mask.

So yes, fewer people will like you. But the ones who do will actually matter.

How to Be Okay With Disapproval

Being intellectually okay with people not liking you is one thing. Actually being emotionally okay with it is another. Here's how to get there:

1. Recognize that disapproval is inevitable: No matter what you do, someone will disapprove. Might as well be disapproved of for being yourself than for being a watered-down version nobody actually connects with.

2. Question whose approval you're seeking: Whose opinion actually matters to you? Whose values align with yours? Whose judgment you respect? Everyone else's opinion is just noise.

3. Remember that their dislike says more about them: People's reactions to you are filtered through their own experiences, insecurities, and biases. Their dislike often has very little to do with you and a lot to do with their stuff.

4. Get comfortable with being misunderstood: Not everyone will understand you. Not everyone will get what you're about. That's okay. You're not here to be universally understood. You're here to live your life.

5. Practice tolerating the discomfort: When someone doesn't like you, it feels bad. Sit with that discomfort. Feel it. Notice that it doesn't actually kill you. The feeling passes. You survive.

The more you practice being disliked and surviving it, the less power it has over you. The fear of disapproval loses its grip when you've actually experienced disapproval and lived through it.

The Different Types of Disapproval

Not all disapproval is created equal. Some you should care about. Some you should ignore entirely.

Disapproval from people you respect: If someone whose values align with yours, whose judgment you trust, whose opinion matters to you expresses concern or disapproval, listen. Maybe they're seeing something you're not.

This doesn't mean you have to change. But it's worth considering their perspective.

Disapproval from people whose values don't align with yours: If someone who represents everything you don't want to be disapproves of you, congratulations. You're on the right track.

Their disapproval is confirmation that you're not becoming them. That's good news.

Disapproval rooted in projection or insecurity: Sometimes people don't like you because you're doing something they wish they could do but can't. Or because you represent a threat to their worldview. Or because your success makes them uncomfortable with their lack thereof.

That's not about you. That's about them. Ignore it.

Disapproval for setting boundaries: When you start having boundaries, people who benefited from your lack of boundaries will disapprove. Let them. Their disapproval is confirmation that your boundaries are working.

The Freedom in Not Being Liked

When you release yourself from the need to be universally liked, you get your life back.

You can:

• Express opinions without constantly hedging

- Make choices based on what you want, not what others will approve of
- Set boundaries without guilt
- Be weird, quirky, yourself
- Pursue goals that others don't understand
- Say no without over-explaining
- Exist without performing

You stop spending energy on managing everyone's perception of you. You stop contorting yourself to fit their expectations. You stop shrinking to make others comfortable.

And all that energy you were wasting on trying to be liked? You get to use it for actually living.

When Disapproval Hurts (And How to Handle It)

Let's be real: even when you know intellectually that you can't be liked by everyone, it still stings when someone doesn't like you.

Especially if:

- It's someone you care about or hoped to connect with
- It's a whole group rejecting you
- It's public or humiliating
- It confirms an insecurity you already have
- It comes from someone whose opinion you value

It's okay to feel hurt. You're human. Rejection hurts. Disapproval stings. That doesn't mean you're doing something wrong. It just means you're human.

How to process it:

Feel it: Don't suppress the hurt. Don't pretend it doesn't matter. Feel disappointed. Feel sad. Feel hurt. Then let it process through.

Reality check: Is their disapproval actually about you, or about their stuff? Are they disapproving of something real, or something they projected onto you?

Values check: Do you respect their opinion? Do their values align with yours? If not, why does their disapproval matter?

Support check: Talk to people who do get you. Who do like you. Who see your value. Let them remind you that not everyone's opinion matters equally.

Action check: Is there anything you actually want to change based on this feedback? Or is this just information that you're not their person? If there's nothing to change, file it under 'not everyone will like me' and move on.

The People Who Matter

Here's the thing: you don't need everyone to like you. You need the right people to like you. The people whose values align with yours. The people who see you and appreciate you. The people who connect with the real you, not the performed version.

Focus your energy there. On deepening connections with people who actually get you. On being more yourself with people who appreciate that. On building relationships with people whose approval actually matters because you respect and value them too.

Stop wasting energy trying to win over people who were never going to be your people anyway. Stop performing for audiences who don't even see you. Stop sacrificing yourself for approval that won't fulfil you even if you get it.

The right people will like you without you having to work for it. They'll appreciate your authenticity, not your performance. They'll value your boundaries, not punish you for them. They'll like you more when you're yourself, not less.

Those are your people. Focus there.

The Permission You Need

You have permission to:

- Be disliked
- Disappoint people
- Not be everyone's cup of tea
- Be polarizing
- Have opinions that others disagree with
- Make choices others wouldn't make
- Be fully yourself even when it means some people won't like you

You're not here to be universally liked. You're here to live your life. To be yourself. To connect deeply with people who appreciate the real you. To build a life that actually fulfils you, not one that earns the most approval.

So let go of the fantasy of universal approval. It's exhausting, impossible, and hollow even if you achieve it.

Instead, pursue authenticity. Pursue genuine connection with people who matter. Pursue a life that's actually yours, not one designed to earn approval from people whose opinions you don't even respect.

It's okay if they don't like you. Really. It's okay.

PART FOUR

WORKPLACE DYNAMICS

Chapter 13: Your Boss Is Not Your Parent (Stop Treating Them Like One)

You're doing it again. Seeking approval from your boss like you're still trying to earn your parent's love. Working overtime to prove your worth. Feeling devastated when they criticize you. Organizing your whole emotional state around whether they're pleased with you.

Your boss is not your parent. They're your boss. And the sooner you stop confusing the two, the healthier your work life will be.

This chapter is about recognizing when you're bringing your family dynamics into the workplace and learning to have a professional relationship with authority figures instead of reenacting childhood trauma.

The Parent-Boss Confusion

If you had parents whose approval was hard to earn, you probably unconsciously recreate that dynamic with your boss. You:

- Work excessive hours trying to prove your worth
- Feel crushed by criticism, even constructive feedback
- Need constant reassurance that you're doing well
- Can't separate your self-worth from your job performance
- Feel like you owe your boss loyalty beyond what's professional
- Struggle to set boundaries because it feels like disappointing a parent
- Take their moods personally

- Desperately want their approval and praise

This isn't about whether your boss is a good boss or a bad boss. This is about you projecting parental dynamics onto a professional relationship.

Your boss is paying you to do a job. That's the relationship. They're not raising you. They're not validating your worth as a human. They're managing your performance at work. That's it.

Why You're Seeking Their Approval

If you're constantly seeking your boss's approval, it's probably because you learned that approval from authority figures was:

Conditional: Your parents' love/attention/pride was conditional on your performance. So now you believe your worth at work is also conditional. You have to keep earning it.

Scarce: Praise was rare in your family. When you got it, it felt amazing. So now you're chasing that high at work, constantly working harder to get that rare moment of approval.

Tied to your identity: Your parents made your achievements about their pride, not your growth. So now when your boss is pleased, you feel valuable. When they're not, you feel worthless.

A measure of safety: If your parents were unpredictable or volatile, you learned to monitor their moods closely for safety. Now you're doing the same with your boss. Reading their mood, adjusting your behaviour, trying to keep them happy so you feel safe.

But here's the thing: your boss's approval doesn't actually mean what you think it means. Getting praise from your boss doesn't make you worthy. Getting criticism doesn't make you worthless. It's just feedback about work performance. That's all.

The Good Child at Work

If you were the 'good child' in your family, you're probably the 'good employee' at work. The one who:

- Never says no to extra work
- Stays late without being asked
- Takes on everyone else's responsibilities
- Never complains or pushes back
- Makes yourself indispensable
- Burns out regularly but keeps going

You learned that being 'good' meant being easy, compliant, and high-achieving. You learned that your value came from being useful. You learned that having needs or boundaries made you difficult.

So now you're that person at work. The one everyone can rely on because you never say no. The one who gets piled with extra work because 'you're so good at handling things.' The one who's exhausted and resentful but keeps smiling.

And your boss loves this. Of course they do. You're the perfect employee. From their perspective. You work for free, you don't complain, you don't ask for raises, you just keep delivering.

But this isn't sustainable. And it's not healthy. And it's definitely not what you owe them.

When Criticism Feels Like Rejection

Does criticism from your boss send you into a shame spiral? Do you replay it for days? Does one piece of negative feedback negate all the positive feedback you've ever received?

That's your childhood programming talking.

If criticism from your parents felt like rejection, criticism from your boss will trigger the same response. Your nervous system can't tell the difference between 'your report needs revision' and 'you're a disappointment.'

But here's what's actually happening: your boss is giving you feedback about your work. Not about your worth. Not about whether you're lovable. Just about work.

Learning to separate work feedback from personal rejection is crucial. Here's how:

1. Pause before reacting: When you receive criticism, your first response is probably emotional. That's your childhood wound activating. Take a breath. Wait for the emotional wave to pass before you respond.

2. Separate the feedback from your worth: Remind yourself: 'This is about my work, not about me as a person. I can improve my work without it meaning I'm fundamentally flawed.'

3. Ask clarifying questions: Instead of spiralling, get specific. 'Can you help me understand what specifically needs to change?' This turns vague criticism into actionable feedback.

4. Look for patterns: Is this the first time you're hearing this feedback, or is it a pattern? If it's new, it might just be this one thing. If it's a pattern, there's something to address.

5. Remember your other successes: One piece of critical feedback doesn't erase all your accomplishments. Keep perspective.

Your boss's opinion of your work is important. It affects your job. But it's not the ultimate measure of your value as a human. Remember that.

The Loyalty Trap

Do you feel like you owe your boss loyalty beyond what's professional? Like leaving for a better opportunity would be betraying them? Like you have to put up with poor treatment because they 'took a chance on you'?

That's parent-child thinking.

Your boss didn't do you a favour by hiring you. They hired you because you were qualified and they needed someone to do the work. It was a mutually beneficial transaction. You don't owe them your life.

Loyalty in a professional context means:

- Doing your job well
- Being honest and ethical
- Not sabotaging the company
- Giving appropriate notice when you leave

Loyalty does NOT mean:

- Staying in a job that underpays you
- Accepting poor treatment
- Sacrificing your health or personal life
- Turning down better opportunities
- Working for free
- Never setting boundaries

Your company would replace you within weeks if you left. Remember that when you're feeling guilty about prioritizing yourself.

Setting Boundaries With Your Boss

If you've been treating your boss like a parent whose approval you need, setting boundaries is going to feel terrifying. It's going to feel like rebellion. Like disrespect. Like you're being a bad employee.

You're not. You're being a professional with healthy boundaries.

Healthy work boundaries include:

- Not responding to emails/messages outside work hours (unless that's explicitly part of your job)
- Saying no to additional work when you're at capacity
- Taking your full lunch break
- Using your vacation days
- Leaving on time when your work is done
- Not making yourself available 24/7

• Asking for compensation when asked to do extra work

How to set these boundaries:

Be matter-of-fact: Don't apologize. Don't over-explain. Just state the boundary clearly.

'I'm at capacity right now. I can take this on if we deprioritize X, or we can discuss timelines.'

Offer solutions when appropriate: If you're saying no to something, sometimes it helps to offer an alternative. But you're not required to solve every problem.

'I can't stay late today. I can come in early tomorrow if that works, or Sarah might be able to help.'

Don't ask permission: You're informing them of your limits, not asking if it's okay to have limits.

'I'll be logging off at 6pm and won't be checking email until tomorrow morning.'

Be consistent: If you set a boundary once but then violate it yourself, you've taught them the boundary is negotiable. Be consistent.

When Your Boss Actually Is Like Your Parent

Sometimes your boss isn't just reminding you of your parent. They actually ARE like your parent. They're:

• Critical and impossible to please

• Volatile and unpredictable

• Taking credit for your work

• Playing favourites

- Manipulative and controlling
- Boundary-violating

In this case, you're not just projecting. You've actually found yourself working for someone who triggers your old wounds because they're exhibiting similar patterns.

This is more complicated because:

- Your emotional responses are both triggered AND appropriate
- You need boundaries AND they probably won't respect them
- The situation is actually harmful AND you're also bringing your own baggage

If your boss is actually toxic (we'll cover this more in the next chapter), you might need to:

- Document everything
- Build an exit strategy
- Protect yourself emotionally while you're there
- Work on not internalizing their treatment

But even with a toxic boss, understanding your parent-boss confusion helps. It helps you separate what's their dysfunction and what's your triggered response. Both can be true.

Redefining Professional Success

If you've been measuring your worth by your boss's approval, you need a new metric for success. One that's actually within your control.

Better measures of professional success:

- Are you learning and growing in your role?
- Are you being compensated fairly?
- Are you maintaining work-life balance?
- Are you meeting your own standards of quality?
- Are you building skills that serve your career goals?
- Are you being treated with respect?

Notice these are all about you, not about what your boss thinks of you.

Your boss's opinion matters for practical reasons. It affects your reviews, your raises, your job security. But it shouldn't be the core of your self-worth.

You're not their child seeking approval. You're a professional providing labour in exchange for compensation. Remember the actual nature of the relationship.

The Exit Option

Here's something you couldn't do as a child with your parents: leave.

You're an adult now. If this job isn't working for you, you can leave. You're not trapped. You're not obligated to stay. You don't owe them years of loyalty for hiring you.

Knowing you can leave changes everything. It shifts the power dynamic. It reminds you that this is a voluntary professional relationship, not an inescapable family bond.

You don't have to leave. But knowing you could? That's freedom.

Use that knowledge. Make decisions from a place of 'I'm choosing to be here' rather than 'I'm trapped here.' It changes how you show up.

What a Healthy Boss Relationship Looks Like

A healthy boss-employee relationship is:

- Professional, not parental
- Transactional at its core (you provide work, they provide compensation)
- Based on clear expectations and feedback
- Respectful of boundaries
- Focused on performance, not worth as a person
- Collaborative without being enmeshed

Your boss should:

- Give you clear expectations
- Provide constructive feedback
- Recognize good work
- Respect your time and boundaries
- Compensate you fairly
- Treat you professionally

Your boss should NOT:

- Be your friend, therapist, or parent
- Have access to all your time and energy
- Make you feel worthless as a person
- Violate your boundaries regularly
- Expect unlimited loyalty and sacrifice

If you're getting the second list instead of the first, it might be time to start looking for the exit.

The Work You Need to Do

Separating your boss from your parent requires conscious effort:

• Notice when you're seeking approval beyond what's professional

• Catch yourself when criticism triggers shame spirals

• Recognize when you're working extra hours to prove your worth

• Identify when loyalty feelings are about childhood wounds, not professional ethics

• Practice setting boundaries without feeling like you're being a bad child

This is ongoing work. The pattern is deeply ingrained. But every time you catch it and choose differently, you're building a healthier relationship with authority and with work.

Your boss is not your parent. Your job is not your identity. Your professional performance is not your worth. Work is work.

Remember that.

Chapter 14: The Toxic Boss: A Survival Guide

Let's be clear about what we're talking about here: a toxic boss is not just someone who's demanding or has high standards or occasionally gives critical feedback. A toxic boss is someone who creates a consistently harmful work environment through their behaviour.

They might be:

- Verbally abusive or demeaning
- Unpredictable and volatile
- Taking credit for your work
- Playing employees against each other
- Micromanaging to the point of suffocation
- Setting impossible standards then punishing you for failing
- Violating boundaries consistently
- Creating a culture of fear

If you have a toxic boss, this chapter is your survival guide. Because sometimes you can't immediately leave. Sometimes you need to stay for financial reasons, or until you find something else, or because leaving isn't currently an option.

So here's how to protect yourself while you're there.

Recognizing Toxic Versus Difficult

Not every difficult boss is toxic. Some bosses are just:

- Direct communicators (feels harsh but isn't abusive)

- High-performing with high expectations (demanding but fair)
- Poor managers who are well-meaning but untrained
- Going through their own stress and handling it badly

A difficult boss can be worked with. A toxic boss creates consistent psychological harm.

Signs your boss is actually toxic:

Pattern of abuse: It's not occasional stress. It's a consistent pattern of demeaning, undermining, or abusive behaviour.

Creates fear, not respect: You're afraid of them, not because they have high standards, but because they're unpredictable, vindictive, or cruel.

Violates boundaries systematically: They expect you available 24/7, intrude on your personal life, don't respect reasonable work boundaries.

Takes credit, assigns blame: Your successes become theirs. Your failures are entirely yours. They never take accountability.

Plays favourites and creates divisions: They pit employees against each other, play favourites, create toxic competition.

Gaslights: They deny saying things they said, blame you for their mistakes, make you question your reality.

Retaliates: If you speak up, set a boundary, or challenge them, they punish you through assignments, reviews, or treatment.

If multiple items on that list are true, you have a toxic boss. Not just a difficult one. Actually toxic.

Why You Can't 'Fix' Them

You cannot manage your way out of having a toxic boss. You cannot be so good at your job that they stop being toxic. You cannot set boundaries effectively enough that they respect you.

Because the problem isn't your performance. The problem is their character, their management style, their unhealed wounds, their lack of emotional regulation.

You cannot fix that. You didn't cause it. You can't control it. You can't cure it.

All you can do is protect yourself while you're in proximity to it.

Survival Strategy 1: Document Everything

This is not optional. Document everything.

- Every conversation (follow up with 'just to confirm' emails)
- Every assignment and deadline
- Every incident of abusive behaviour
- Every time they change expectations
- Every time they take credit for your work
- Every promise they make and break

How to document:

Email yourself: After meetings or conversations, email yourself a summary with the date and what was discussed.

Paper trail: Confirm verbal conversations in writing: 'Just to confirm our conversation, you said X and the deadline is Y.'

Save everything: Keep copies of your work, emails, performance reviews, everything. Not on your work computer. Use personal storage.

Note dates and witnesses: When documenting incidents, note the date, time, location, who was present, what was said.

Why this matters: If things escalate, if you need to go to HR, if you need to protect yourself legally, you'll need documentation. Your memory isn't enough. Get it in writing.

Survival Strategy 2: Emotional Detachment

This is the hardest part: you have to emotionally detach from your toxic boss's opinion of you.

Their criticism? Not about you. Their anger? Not about you. Their impossible standards? Not about you. It's about them. Their dysfunction. Their issues. Their lack of emotional regulation.

How to practice detachment:

Remind yourself of the truth: 'This person is dysfunctional. Their opinion doesn't define my worth or my abilities.'

Observe, don't absorb: When they're raging or criticizing, imagine you're a scientist observing behaviour. 'Interesting. They're having a disproportionate response again.' Don't internalize it.

Separate feedback into categories: Is there any legitimate work feedback buried in the toxicity? Extract that. Discard the rest.

Don't seek their approval: You will not get it, or you'll get it unpredictably, which is worse. Stop trying. Do your job competently and get your validation elsewhere.

Gray rock when possible: Give them nothing to work with emotionally. Be boring. Professional. Neutral. Don't feed their need for drama or reaction.

This doesn't mean you won't feel the impact. You will. But emotional detachment means not making their dysfunction about you.

Survival Strategy 3: Boundary Enforcement (Carefully)

With a toxic boss, boundary enforcement is tricky. They don't respect boundaries. But you still need them.

The goal is to set boundaries without making yourself a target.

Pick your battles: You can't enforce every boundary with a toxic boss. Choose the ones that matter most to your wellbeing.

Frame boundaries professionally: Not 'I need work-life balance' but 'I'm not available after 7pm. I can address this first thing in the morning.'

Be strategic about timing: Don't set boundaries when they're already angry or volatile. Wait for a calmer moment.

Document boundary violations: When they violate a boundary, document it. This might matter later.

Have consequences ready: You might not be able to leave, but you can have smaller consequences. Stop checking email at night. Stop taking on extra work. Stop engaging beyond what's required.

Know that they might retaliate. That's the risk. Which is why you pick your battles carefully and document everything.

Survival Strategy 4: Build Your Exit Strategy

Even if you can't leave right now, start building your exit strategy today.

- Update your resume
- Start networking
- Build marketable skills
- Save money
- Research other opportunities
- Connect with recruiters in your field
- Work on your LinkedIn profile
- Start looking, even if you're not ready to leave yet

Why? Because knowing you're building an exit changes how you feel about being there. You're not trapped. You're choosing to stay for now while building your way out.

That mental shift, from trapped to strategic, matters for your mental health.

Survival Strategy 5: Find Support Outside Work

Don't try to survive this alone. You need:

A therapist: If you can afford it, get one. Processing the impact of a toxic work environment with a professional is invaluable.

Trusted friends/family: People who will validate your reality when your boss is gaslighting you. People who will remind you that you're not crazy.

Peer support: Other people who've dealt with toxic bosses. They get it in ways others don't.

Activities outside work: Things that remind you that work isn't your whole life. Hobbies, relationships, interests that have nothing to do with your job.

Don't isolate. That makes it worse. Connect with people who see your worth, even when your boss doesn't.

Survival Strategy 6: Protect Your Mental Health

Working for a toxic boss takes a toll on your mental health. Protect it aggressively:

- Take all your vacation days
- Use sick days for mental health if needed
- Set hard boundaries around work hours when possible
- Don't take work home (mentally or physically) if you can avoid it
- Exercise, sleep, eat well. Basic self-care isn't optional

• Consider medication if anxiety/depression become unmanageable

• Have a decompression ritual after work (shower, walk, whatever helps you transition out of work mode)

You cannot be your best self in a toxic environment. Stop expecting that of yourself. Surviving is enough.

When to Go to HR (And When Not To)

HR is not your friend. HR protects the company, not you. Remember that.

But sometimes, going to HR is the right move:

When to go to HR:

• You have clear documentation of illegal behaviour (discrimination, harassment, retaliation)

• You've tried addressing issues directly and been retaliated against

• The behaviour is severe and creating a hostile work environment

• You have witnesses and documentation

• You're prepared for possible retaliation and have an exit strategy

When NOT to go to HR:

• You don't have documentation

• It's your word against theirs

• The toxic boss is protected by higher-ups

• You're not prepared to leave if it goes badly

• HR has a history of protecting bad managers

If you do go to HR:

- Bring documentation
- Be factual, not emotional
- Focus on behaviour and impact, not your feelings
- Have specific examples with dates
- Know what outcome you're requesting
- Be prepared for nothing to change
- Be prepared for retaliation

The Reality Check

Here are some hard truths:

Your toxic boss might never face consequences. They might continue to be promoted. They might continue to harm others. Justice might not happen.

You staying and trying to change things probably won't work. Unless you're in a position of power or the company cares about these issues, your efforts will likely be futile.

The best outcome is usually: you leave. Not because you failed. But because protecting yourself is more important than trying to fix a broken system.

Leaving isn't giving up. Leaving is choosing yourself. Leaving is recognizing that your mental health and career are more valuable than trying to make a dysfunctional situation functional.

How to Know When It Is Time to Go

You should leave when:

- The job is affecting your physical health (chronic stress, illness, sleep problems)
- The job is affecting your mental health (anxiety, depression, trauma responses)
- You dread going to work every single day
- You're becoming a person you don't like (bitter, cynical, mean)
- The toxicity is affecting your personal relationships
- You've lost all ability to feel accomplishment or pride in your work
- You can't remember why you used to like this field
- You're staying only out of fear, not for any positive reason

If several of those are true, start actively looking. Don't wait until you're completely broken.

What You Owe Them (Nothing)

You don't owe a toxic boss:

- Two weeks notice (if leaving would harm you)
- An explanation for why you're leaving
- Fixing all your projects before you go
- Training your replacement
- Maintaining the pretence that everything was fine
- Protecting their reputation

You can choose to do some of these things for your own reasons. Maintaining professional reputation, not burning bridges with colleagues, personal integrity. But you don't owe them to your toxic boss.

Do what protects you. That's what matters.

After You Leave

When you finally get out, you might be surprised by:

- How much damage was done that you didn't realize while you were in it
- How long it takes to recover
- How your nervous system stays on high alert
- How you second-guess yourself at your new job
- How angry you are once you're safe enough to feel it

This is normal. Working for a toxic boss is traumatic. Give yourself time and space to heal. Consider therapy specifically for workplace trauma.

And know this: you survived. You got out. You chose yourself. That's worth celebrating.

Chapter 15: Stop Working for Free

You're doing it. Right now. Working for free.

Answering emails at 10pm. Taking work calls on your day off. Staying late without compensation. Working through lunch. Doing tasks outside your job description. Being available 24/7.

And nobody's paying you for it.

This chapter is about recognizing when you're giving away your labour for free and learning to stop.

How You're Working for Free

Let's count the ways:

Unpaid overtime: If you're salaried, you might think overtime is expected. It's not. Salary means a set number of hours. Anything beyond that is free labour you're volunteering.

Off-hours availability: Checking email after hours. Taking calls on weekends. Being 'on call' without on-call pay. That's work. You're working. For free.

Working through breaks: Lunch breaks are legally required. If you're working through them, you're working for free.

Scope creep: You were hired for X, but now you're also doing Y and Z. Those additional responsibilities should come with additional compensation. If they don't, you're working for free.

Unpaid 'favours': 'Can you just quickly...' adds up. Each 'quick favour' is work you're not being paid for.

Training others: Training new employees might be part of your job. But if you're regularly training people and it's not in your job description, that's work you're not being compensated for.

Add it up. How many hours a week are you working without compensation? 5? 10? 20? That's free labour you're giving your employer.

Why You're Doing It

You're working for free because:

You think it's expected: Everyone else seems to be doing it, so you assume it's part of the job. But just because it's normalized doesn't mean it's okay.

You're afraid of being seen as lazy: If you only work your contracted hours, you worry you'll be seen as not a team player, not committed, not dedicated.

You're trying to prove your worth: You think working extra hours will lead to recognition, raises, promotions. Sometimes it does. Often it just leads to more work.

You feel guilty saying no: When someone asks you to stay late or handle something over the weekend, saying no feels wrong. You've been trained to be accommodating.

You're scared of losing your job: If you don't go above and beyond, someone else will, and you'll be replaced. That fear keeps you working for free.

All of these reasons are understandable. None of them justify working for free.

The Cost of Free Labor

What are you actually losing by working for free?

Money: Let's do the math. If you make $50,000/year for 40 hours/week, that's about $24/hour. If you're working an extra 10 hours/week unpaid, that's $240/week, or $12,480/year. You're giving your employer $12,480 of free labour annually.

That's real money. Money you could be earning. Money you could be saving. Money you could be using to live your life.

Time: Every hour you work for free is an hour you're not spending on yourself, your relationships, your hobbies, your rest. That time is gone. You don't get it back.

Energy: Working extra hours depletes you. You have less energy for your personal life. Less patience for your loved ones. Less capacity for joy.

Leverage: When you work for free, you teach your employer that you'll do it. You lose your leverage to negotiate for fair compensation because they know you'll just do it anyway.

Self-respect: Every time you work for free, you're telling yourself that your time isn't valuable. That you don't deserve to be compensated fairly. That's damaging.

The 'But Everyone Else Does It' Trap

Yes, everyone else might be working for free too. That doesn't make it okay. It just means everyone is being exploited.

Companies love to normalize unpaid overtime. They love to create cultures where working 50-60 hour weeks is seen as standard. Because it means they get significantly more labour than they're paying for.

But you don't have to participate in that just because others are.

Someone has to be the first to set a boundary. It might as well be you.

How to Stop Working for Free

Here's how to reclaim your time and stop volunteering free labour:

1. Know your actual job: What are you actually contracted to do? What hours are you actually being paid for? Get clear on this.

2. Track your hours: For one week, track exactly how many hours you're working. Including email time, calls, 'quick tasks.' See the real number.

3. Set boundaries around work hours: Decide what hours you're willing to work. Stick to them. Don't check email outside those hours. Don't take calls. Be unavailable.

4. Say no to scope creep: When asked to take on additional responsibilities: 'I'm at capacity with my current role. If this is a priority, what should I deprioritize? Or can we discuss adjusting my compensation to reflect these additional duties?'

5. Charge for your time: If you're asked to work outside hours: 'I can do this during work hours tomorrow, or if it's urgent and needs to happen tonight, I'll need overtime compensation.'

6. Take your breaks: Full lunch break. Coffee breaks. Actually take them. Don't work through them.

7. Leave on time: When your work hours end, leave. If someone tries to grab you with 'just one quick thing' on your way out: 'I'll address this first thing tomorrow.'

The Scripts You Need

Here are specific phrases for specific situations:

For after-hours emails: 'I'm not available after [time]. I'll respond to this tomorrow during work hours.'

For weekend work: 'I'm not available on weekends. I can prioritize this Monday morning.'

For additional responsibilities: 'I'm at capacity. If you'd like me to take this on, let's discuss which of my current responsibilities I should deprioritize, or we can discuss adjusting my role and compensation.'

For urgent requests at end of day: 'I'm leaving for the day. If this is truly urgent, let's discuss overtime compensation. Otherwise, I'll handle it first thing tomorrow.'

For working through lunch: 'I'm taking my lunch break. I'll be back at [time].'

Notice: no apologies. No extensive explanations. Just clear boundaries about when you're working and when you're not.

What If They Push Back?

They probably will push back. Here's how to handle it:

'But we need this done now': 'I understand the urgency. My work hours are [X]. I can prioritize this tomorrow, or if it needs to be done tonight, let's discuss overtime compensation.'

'This is just how it is here': 'I'm willing to work the hours I'm contracted for. If the role requires regular overtime, that should be reflected in the compensation.'

'Everyone else does it': 'I'm setting boundaries around my work hours. This is what works for me.'

'You're not a team player': 'I'm happy to be a team player during my work hours. What I do outside those hours is my personal time.'

'We can't afford overtime pay': 'Then the work will need to be done during regular hours, or we can discuss prioritization.'

Stand firm. They're used to people caving. Don't.

When It Is Actually Part of Your Job

Some jobs legitimately require flexibility:

- On-call doctors, emergency services
- Roles explicitly requiring availability (with on-call pay)
- High-level positions with explicit after-hours expectations

But even in these roles:

- You should be compensated appropriately
- The expectations should be explicit in your contract
- There should still be boundaries and limits

If you're expected to be available 24/7, you should be paid like you're available 24/7. If you're not, you're being exploited.

The Promotion Carrot

'If you just work hard enough, you'll get promoted.' Maybe. Or maybe you'll just be expected to keep working that hard forever.

Here's what actually happens: You work 60 hours a week hoping for a promotion. You get the promotion. Now you're expected to work 60 hours a week in your new role because that's what they know you'll do.

The bar just gets raised. The expectation just gets higher. You never actually get to stop overworking.

Don't sacrifice your life for a promotion that might never come. And if it does come, set boundaries from the start of the new role.

The Worst Case Scenario

What's the worst that could happen if you stop working for free?

- They could be unhappy with you
- You might not get a raise/promotion this cycle
- You might be seen as not a 'go-getter'
- They could even fire you

Let's address that last one: if they fire you for refusing to work for free, that's information about that company. They were exploiting you. Getting fired from an exploitative situation isn't failure. It's a forced exit from something that was harming you.

And honestly? Most companies won't fire you for setting reasonable boundaries. They'll grumble. They'll push back. But ultimately, if you're good at your job during your actual work hours, most won't fire you for not volunteering free labour.

The risk is smaller than you think.

What You're Worth

Your time has value. Your expertise has value. Your labour has value. If a company wants access to your time, expertise, and labour, they need to compensate you for it. That's how employment works. You trade your labour for money.

When you work for free, you're giving away something valuable. You're being charitable to a for-profit entity that wouldn't extend the same charity to you.

Stop.

Know your worth. Charge for your time. Set boundaries. Leave on time. Take your breaks. Say no to free labour.

You're not a volunteer. You're an employee. Act accordingly.

Chapter 16: Their Disorganization Is Not Your Emergency

Your coworker forgot about a deadline. Your boss waited until the last minute. Your client didn't get you information when they said they would. And now it's an emergency. And somehow, it's your job to fix it. By staying late. By rearranging your priorities. By sacrificing your evening/weekend/sanity.

No.

Their poor planning is not your emergency. Their disorganization is not your crisis to solve. Their failure to manage their time doesn't create an obligation for you to sacrifice yours.

This chapter is about stopping the pattern of making other people's disorganization your problem.

How This Pattern Works

Someone else fails to plan appropriately. They create a crisis through their own lack of organization, procrastination, or poor time management. Then they expect you to drop everything and fix it.

And you do. Because:

- You don't want to let the team down
- You feel guilty saying no to 'emergencies'
- You're worried about being seen as not a team player
- You've been trained to accommodate others
- You feel responsible for problems that aren't yours

So you stay late. You rearrange your schedule. You sacrifice your plans. You fix their crisis.

And what do they learn? That if they don't plan, you'll bail them out. So they keep not planning. And you keep bailing them out. The cycle continues.

The Different Types of Manufactured Emergencies

The Chronic Procrastinator: This person always waits until the last minute. Every project becomes an emergency because they didn't start until the deadline was tomorrow.

They've learned that procrastinating works because someone (you) will always help them scramble at the end.

The Poor Planner: This person consistently underestimates how long things take, doesn't account for potential problems, doesn't build in buffer time.

Every project becomes a crisis because they didn't plan realistically.

The Last-Minute Person: This person sits on information, doesn't communicate needs early, then dumps everything on you at the last possible moment.

'I meant to tell you earlier, but...' creates urgency where there didn't need to be any.

The Disorganized Boss: This person doesn't manage their workload, doesn't prioritize effectively, doesn't plan ahead. Then their chaos becomes your emergency.

'I know I told you that was due next week, but actually I need it tomorrow.'

The Chaos Creator: This person thrives on drama and urgency. They create crises where none exist because they like the adrenaline or the attention.

Everything is always urgent with them. Nothing can wait. It's all an emergency.

Why It Is Not Actually Your Emergency

Just because someone else has an emergency doesn't mean you have an emergency.

Their crisis was created by their choices:

- They chose to procrastinate
- They chose not to plan adequately
- They chose not to communicate earlier
- They chose not to manage their time

Those were their choices. The consequences are theirs to manage.

You didn't create this crisis. You're not responsible for solving it. Their emergency is not automatically your emergency.

How to Stop Rescuing Them

1. Don't make their emergency yours: When someone comes to you with a last-minute crisis, your first response doesn't have to be 'how can I fix this?' It can be 'what's your plan for addressing this?'

Put the responsibility back on them. They created it. They need to solve it.

2. Set realistic expectations about your availability: 'I'm at capacity today. I can help with this tomorrow afternoon.'

You're not refusing to help. You're setting a timeline that works for you. If their emergency can't wait until tomorrow, that's information about whether it's actually your problem.

3. Stop rewarding poor planning: Every time you drop everything to fix someone's crisis, you teach them that poor planning works. Stop teaching them that.

Let them experience the natural consequences of their disorganization. Maybe they'll learn to plan better.

4. Distinguish real emergencies from manufactured ones: Real emergency: The server crashed. Someone was hospitalized. There's a genuine crisis that couldn't have been predicted.

Manufactured emergency: Someone forgot about a deadline. Someone didn't start until the last minute. Someone changed their mind at the last second.

Real emergencies warrant flexibility. Manufactured ones don't.

5. Offer help on your terms: 'I can't stay late, but I can spend 30 minutes helping you prioritize tomorrow morning.'

You're not refusing to help. You're helping in a way that doesn't require you to sacrifice your boundaries.

The Scripts You Need

When someone dumps a crisis on you: 'That sounds stressful. What's your plan for handling it?'

Notice: you're not offering to fix it. You're asking what they plan to do about it.

When asked to stay late for their emergency: 'I have plans this evening. I can help with this during work hours tomorrow.'

Your plans don't have to be elaborate. They can be 'rest' or 'dinner' or 'nothing.' They're still plans. They still matter.

When someone's poor planning affects your timeline: 'I understand this is urgent for you. My current priorities are X and Y. If you need me to prioritize this instead, which of those should I deprioritize?'

Make them make the trade-off explicit. Make them acknowledge that adding something urgent means something else gets pushed.

When the crisis is due to lack of communication: 'I needed this information last week to meet the deadline. I can get this done by [realistic date], or if you need it sooner, you'll need to assign it to someone else.'

Don't let their failure to communicate early become your problem to solve through overwork.

When someone repeatedly creates emergencies: 'I've noticed this has happened several times. Going forward, I need [X amount of notice] to be able to help. Last-minute requests won't be possible.'

Set expectations explicitly. Stop accommodating the pattern.

When Your Boss Is the Problem

This is trickier when it's your boss who's disorganized and creating emergencies.

You can't always say 'that's not my problem' to your boss. But you can:

Ask clarifying questions: 'To meet this timeline, I'll need to deprioritize X and Y. Is that okay, or should we discuss timeline adjustments?'

Make the trade-offs visible. Force them to acknowledge what's being sacrificed to accommodate their disorganization.

Suggest process improvements: 'I've noticed we often have tight turnarounds. Would it help if we had a weekly planning meeting to get ahead of deadlines?'

Sometimes disorganized bosses just need better systems. Offering to help create those systems can reduce the crisis cycle.

Set boundaries where you can: 'I can get this done by [realistic time], but not sooner without sacrificing quality. Which would you prefer?'

Give them choices. Sometimes rushing isn't actually necessary if they realize it means lower quality.

Document the pattern: If your boss's disorganization is consistent and affecting your work-life balance, document it. Note the times, the requests, the lack of planning. This might be relevant for HR or future reviews.

The Team Player Trap

'But we need to be team players!' Yes. During work hours. For legitimate emergencies. With reasonable notice when possible.

Being a team player doesn't mean:

- Sacrificing your personal time regularly
- Accommodating poor planning consistently
- Making other people's disorganization your emergency
- Never saying no
- Working for free to fix problems you didn't create

Being a team player means:

- Doing your job well
- Communicating clearly
- Helping when you reasonably can
- Collaborating effectively
- Occasionally being flexible for real emergencies

You can be a team player with boundaries. The two aren't mutually exclusive.

What About Genuine Emergencies?

Real emergencies happen. Things outside anyone's control. Actual crises.

In those cases, being flexible makes sense. Helping out makes sense. Going above and beyond makes sense.

But here's the thing: if everything is an emergency, nothing is. If you're constantly dealing with 'emergencies,' they're not emergencies. They're poor planning disguised as urgency.

Real emergencies are rare. They're genuine crises that couldn't have been anticipated or prevented. They're not the same as 'my boss forgot to plan.'

Learn to distinguish. Be flexible for real emergencies. Hold boundaries for manufactured ones.

Breaking the Rescue Cycle

If you've been consistently bailing people out, breaking that pattern will be uncomfortable:

They'll be upset: They've come to rely on you fixing their crises. When you stop, they'll push back.

Let them. Their feelings about your boundaries aren't your problem to fix.

There will be consequences: When you stop rescuing them, their crisis might not get solved. The deadline might be missed. The project might fail.

Those are natural consequences of their poor planning. They need to experience them to learn.

You'll feel guilty: You've been trained to fix things. Not fixing will trigger guilt.

Feel it. Don't act on it. The guilt will pass. Your boundary stays.

Some people will learn: Once they realize you won't bail them out, some people will start planning better. They'll communicate earlier. They'll manage their time.

That's the goal. Teach them that crises don't work with you.

Some won't: Some people won't change. They'll just find someone else to rescue them. Or they'll keep creating crises and dealing with the consequences.

Not your problem. You've set your boundary. What they do with that is up to them.

The Long-Term Benefit

When you stop making other people's disorganization your emergency:

- You get your time back
- You stop working for free
- You teach people to respect your boundaries
- You reduce stress and burnout
- You model healthy boundaries for others
- People learn to plan better (or at least stop expecting you to fix their crises)

It's uncomfortable at first. But it's worth it.

Your Permission

You have permission to:

- Not fix every crisis
- Say no to last-minute emergencies that aren't yours
- Let people experience the consequences of their poor planning
- Prioritize your own time and boundaries
- Be unavailable for manufactured emergencies
- Stop rescuing people from their own disorganization

Their crisis is not your emergency. Say it with me: Their crisis is not your emergency.

You're not responsible for fixing problems you didn't create. You're not obligated to sacrifice your time for someone else's poor planning. You're not required to make their disorganization your priority.

So stop. Set the boundary. Hold it. Let them figure it out.

Their disorganization is not your emergency

Chapter 12: When Friendships Need to End (And How to Let Them Go)

Not all friendships are meant to last forever. Some friendships have a season. Some outgrow their purpose. Some become toxic. Some were never healthy to begin with.

And yet, we're taught that ending friendships is failure. That good people maintain relationships no matter what. That if a friendship ends, someone did something wrong.

That's not true. Sometimes the healthiest thing you can do is let a friendship go. Not because anyone's evil. Not because there was a big dramatic fight. Just because the friendship is no longer serving either of you.

This chapter is about recognizing when friendships need to end and how to release them with grace.

Signs a Friendship Has Run Its Course

How do you know when it's time to let a friendship go?

You feel drained, not energized: Spending time with this friend consistently leaves you feeling worse, not better. You're exhausted after hanging out. You dread their calls. You feel like you need to recover after seeing them.

Good friendships energize you, even when you're having serious conversations or supporting each other through hard times. If this friendship consistently depletes you, that's a sign.

It's consistently one-sided: You're always the one reaching out, making plans, checking in, giving support. And when you stop initiating, the friendship disappears. That's not a friendship. That's you volunteering at someone else's emotional support centre.

Real friendships are reciprocal over time. Not perfectly equal every single moment, but balanced in the long run. If it's been one-sided for months or years, it's not going to change.

You can't be yourself: You're constantly performing around this friend. Editing yourself. Hiding parts of your personality. Avoiding topics they don't approve of. Walking on eggshells.

Friendships should be places where you can be authentic. If you can't be yourself, what's the point?

They don't respect your boundaries: You've stated clear boundaries. They violate them repeatedly. They test them. They make you feel guilty for having them. They ignore them entirely.

Friendships require mutual respect. If they can't respect your boundaries, they don't respect you. Full stop.

The friendship is based on history, not present connection: You're only friends because you've been friends for a long time. Or because you went through something together years ago. But there's no real connection in the present. You have nothing in common anymore. You don't actually enjoy each other's company.

Shared history is meaningful. But it's not enough to sustain a friendship on its own. If the only thing keeping you connected is the past, it might be time to let go.

They're actively harmful: They gossip about you. They undermine you. They're jealous of your success. They make you feel bad about yourself. They're cruel disguised as 'honest.' They're competitive in unhealthy ways.

Some friendships are actively toxic. If this person consistently makes your life worse, it's not a friendship worth maintaining.

You've grown in different directions: You're not the same people you were when you became friends. Your values have changed. Your lifestyles have changed. Your priorities have changed. And there's no longer alignment.

This isn't anyone's fault. People grow. Sometimes you grow apart. That's okay. It doesn't mean the friendship was meaningless. It just means it's reached its end.

The Different Types of Friendship Endings

Not all friendship endings look the same. Different situations require different approaches.

The Slow Fade: You gradually decrease contact until you're essentially not friends anymore. This works best for friendships that have naturally run their course without major conflict.

How it looks: Stop initiating plans. Take longer to respond to messages. Be less available. Eventually, the friendship just... fades. No drama. No announcement. Just gentle distance.

This is appropriate when: The friendship has been in decline for a while, there's no major conflict, and both of you are kind of over it but nobody wants to make it official.

The Direct Conversation: You explicitly tell them the friendship isn't working for you anymore and you need to step back.

How it looks: 'I've been thinking about our friendship and I don't think it's healthy for me anymore. I need to take some space.'

This is appropriate when: There's been ongoing issues, they keep violating boundaries, or you need closure. Also appropriate when they're someone who won't take hints and you need to be direct.

The Clean Break: You stop all contact. No explanation. No goodbye. Just done.

How it looks: Block. Delete. Move on. Radio silence.

This is appropriate when: The friendship is toxic or abusive, they've repeatedly violated serious boundaries, or any conversation would just give them ammunition to manipulate you.

The Boundary Reduction: You don't end the friendship completely, but you significantly reduce contact and emotionally divest.

How it looks: You're still technically friends, but you see them rarely, share less, invest less emotional energy.

This is appropriate when: You have shared friend groups or circumstances that make a complete break complicated, but you need distance for your wellbeing.

How to Have the Conversation (If You're Having One)

If you decide to have a direct conversation about ending the friendship, here's how to do it:

Be clear: Don't hedge. Don't soften it so much that they don't understand what you're saying. Be direct about the fact that you're stepping back from the friendship.

'I've realized this friendship isn't healthy for me anymore. I need to take a significant step back.'

Don't JADE: You don't owe them an extensive explanation. You don't need to justify your decision. You don't need to argue about whether your feelings are valid. You don't need to defend yourself.

'This isn't working for me' is sufficient. If you want to say more, you can. But you don't have to.

Expect pushback: They'll probably try to convince you to give them another chance. They'll promise to change. They'll make excuses. They might cry. They might get angry.

Hold your boundary. 'I understand you're upset. My decision stands.'

Don't let it turn into a negotiation: You're not asking for their permission. You're informing them of your decision. This isn't a debate.

If they try to negotiate: 'This isn't a discussion. I've made my decision.'

Be prepared to leave: If it's an in-person conversation, be ready to leave if they won't respect your boundary. If it's a phone conversation, be ready to end the call.

'I'm going to go now. I wish you well.'

The Grief of Letting Go

Even when a friendship is unhealthy, ending it hurts. You're grieving:

- The friendship you hoped it would be
- The person you thought they were
- The history you shared
- The future you imagined together
- The role they played in your life
- The social connections tied to this friendship

That grief is real and valid. Let yourself feel it.

You can grieve a relationship that wasn't good for you. You can miss someone who wasn't healthy to be around. You can feel sad about losing something that needed to be lost.

The grief doesn't mean you made the wrong choice. It just means you're human.

Handling Mutual Friends

One of the hardest parts of ending a friendship is navigating shared friend groups.

Do you tell people what happened? Do you stay silent? Do you avoid group events? Do you expect others to pick sides?

Guidelines:

Don't trash talk: It's tempting to tell everyone why you ended the friendship. Don't. It puts mutual friends in an awkward position and makes you look bad.

If people ask: 'We grew apart' or 'The friendship wasn't healthy for me anymore' is sufficient. Don't give details unless they're your close friend independently of this situation.

Don't expect people to pick sides: Your decision to end the friendship is about you and that person. Other people can maintain relationships with both of you. Don't make them choose.

If someone does pick sides against you: That's information about that relationship too.

Set boundaries about your ex-friend: With close friends, you can ask them not to bring up your ex-friend or share information about you with them.

'I'd appreciate if you didn't share details about my life with [person]. And I'd rather not hear about them either.'

Navigate group events carefully: You might need to skip some events. Or arrive late/leave early to minimize overlap. Or just accept that you'll sometimes be in the same space and be cordial but distant.

Do what protects your peace.

When They Won't Let Go

Sometimes you end a friendship and the other person doesn't accept it. They keep reaching out. They show up places they know you'll be. They text. They try to talk through mutual friends.

Your response:

Don't respond: Every response, even 'please stop contacting me,' is engagement. It teaches them that if they push hard enough, you'll respond.

Complete silence is the strongest message.

Block if necessary: If they won't stop, block them. On everything. Phone, social media, email. Block.

This isn't mean. This is protecting your boundary.

Tell mutual friends: If they're using mutual friends to get messages to you, tell those friends: 'I ended my friendship with [person]. Please don't pass along messages from them.'

Consider escalation: If they're harassing you, stalking you, or threatening you, document everything and consider legal options. This is not okay.

How to Not Go Back

There will be moments of weakness. Moments where you miss them. Moments where you wonder if you overreacted. Moments where you're tempted to reach out.

Don't.

Remember why you left:

- Keep a note in your phone of the reasons you ended the friendship
- When you feel nostalgic, reread it
- Remind yourself: you're not missing who they actually were. You're missing who you hoped they'd be

The pattern won't change. If you go back, you'll just end up leaving again. Save yourself the repeat pain.

Opening Space for New Friendships

When you let go of friendships that aren't serving you, you create space, emotional space, time, energy, for friendships that do.

You can't fill your life with healthy friendships if you're spending all your energy maintaining unhealthy ones. You can't meet your people if you're too exhausted from managing friendships that drain you.

Letting go isn't just about ending what's not working. It's about making room for what could work.

The right people are out there. People who will respect your boundaries. People who will reciprocate. People who will appreciate the real you. People who will energize rather than drain you.

But you won't find them if you're too busy clinging to friendships that ended long before you officially let them go.

The Permission to Let Go

You have permission to:

- End friendships that aren't serving you
- Let go without a big explanation
- Grieve friendships that were unhealthy
- Protect your peace even if it disappoints others
- Choose yourself over maintaining a dying friendship
- Walk away from people who consistently hurt you
- Release friendships that are based only on history

Not all friendships are meant to last forever. Some are seasonal. Some are for a specific purpose. Some are lessons in what you don't want.

Let them go when they're done. Not with bitterness. Not with drama. Just with the recognition that this connection has run its course and it's time to release it.

You deserve friendships that fill you up, not drain you dry. You deserve friends who respect you, reciprocate, and appreciate you. You deserve connections that enhance your life, not detract from it.

But you won't have space for those friendships until you let go of the ones that don't serve you.

So let go. With grace, with gratitude for what was good, and with clear eyes about what wasn't.

Let go.

PART FIVE
LOVE & RELATIONSHIPS

Chapter 17: Love Without Losing Yourself

You've done it before. Met someone amazing and slowly, subtly, completely erased yourself to fit their life. Their preferences became yours. Their friends became your social circle. Their interests became your hobbies. You moulded yourself into whatever they needed, until one day you looked in the mirror and didn't recognize the person staring back.

That's not love. That's self-abandonment with romance packaging.

This chapter is about learning to love someone without losing yourself in the process. About maintaining your identity while building a partnership. About being fully present in a relationship while staying fully yourself.

The Disappearing Act

It starts small. You say you like their favourite band when you're actually indifferent. You skip your weekly dinner with friends because they want to stay in. You stop mentioning your interests because they don't share them. You adjust your opinions to match theirs. You make yourself smaller, quieter, more convenient.

And it feels like love. It feels like compromise. It feels like being a good partner.

But somewhere along the way, you stopped being a person and became an accessory to their life.

Signs you're losing yourself in a relationship:

- You can't remember the last time you did something just for you
- Your hobbies have become their hobbies (or you have no hobbies)
- You've lost touch with your friends
- You check with them before making any decision
- You've stopped expressing opinions that differ from theirs
- You don't know what you want anymore because you're so focused on what they want
- You feel anxious when you're not with them
- Your identity is entirely wrapped up in being their partner
- You've stopped doing things that used to bring you joy
- You feel like you don't know who you are outside this relationship

If several of those are true, you're not in a healthy partnership. You're performing a disappearing act.

Why You Do This

You learned early that love is conditional. That to be loved, you need to be what the other person wants. That your authentic self isn't enough. That love requires transformation, accommodation, self-erasure.

Maybe you watched your mother disappear into marriage. Maybe you learned that keeping the peace meant having no needs. Maybe you discovered that the only way to keep someone was to become whoever they needed.

So now, when you fall in love, you fall into old patterns:

You merge instead of connecting: Instead of two whole people coming together, you dissolve your boundaries and become enmeshed. You lose track of where you end and they begin.

You mistake sacrifice for love: You believe that real love means giving up what you want. That compromise means you always give in. That proving your love requires constant self-abandonment.

You confuse harmony with health: Never fighting seems like a good relationship. But if you never disagree, it's probably because you've stopped having opinions.

You use the relationship to avoid yourself: Being consumed by a relationship is easier than facing your own life, your own goals, your own issues. The relationship becomes a convenient place to hide.

None of this is love. It is fear dressed up as devotion.

What Healthy Love Actually Looks Like

Healthy love is two whole people choosing to share their lives while maintaining their individuality.

In healthy love:

- You have separate interests and support each other's pursuits
- You maintain friendships outside the relationship
- You have alone time without it being a crisis
- You can disagree without it threatening the relationship

- You make decisions together, not by one person always deferring
- You grow as individuals while also growing together
- Your identity includes but isn't entirely defined by the relationship
- You're interdependent, not codependent

Healthy love doesn't require you to shrink. It doesn't demand that you erase yourself. It doesn't punish you for being a whole person with your own thoughts, feelings, preferences, and life.

If your relationship requires you to be less than you are, it's not the right relationship.

Maintaining Your Identity

How do you stay yourself while building a life with someone else?

Keep your interests: Even if they don't share them. Especially if they don't share them. You're allowed to have hobbies they don't participate in. You're allowed to be passionate about things they don't care about.

You don't have to like all the same things. You're not the same person. That's good, not a problem.

Maintain your friendships: Your friends aren't optional just because you're in a relationship. Keep seeing them. Keep making plans. Keep investing in those relationships.

A partner who wants to be your only relationship is waving a red flag, not proving their devotion.

Have alone time: You should be able to be alone without your partner spiralling. And you should want to be alone sometimes without it meaning you don't love them.

Alone time isn't rejection. It's self-care. It's how you stay yourself.

Keep your opinions: You're allowed to disagree. You're allowed to have different perspectives. You're allowed to think differently than your partner.

Agreement on everything is suspicious. It usually means someone's pretending.

Pursue your goals: Your dreams don't become less important because you're in a relationship. Keep working toward them. A good partner supports your goals, not replaces them.

Know yourself: Keep checking in with yourself. What do you want? What do you feel? What matters to you? Don't lose touch with your internal compass just because you're navigating with a partner.

The Balance Between Compromise and Self-Abandonment

Relationships require compromise. But there's a difference between healthy compromise and self-abandonment.

Healthy compromise: Both people give a little. Both people get some of what they want. The compromise feels fair and doesn't consistently favour one person.

Example: You want Italian, they want Mexican. You compromise on Thai. Or you alternate. Italian this week,

Mexican next week. Neither person always gets their way. Neither person always gives in.

Self-abandonment: One person consistently sacrifices their preferences. One person always adjusts. One person's wants and needs are always secondary.

Example: You always watch what they want to watch. You always eat where they want to eat. You always do what they want to do. Your preferences don't even enter the conversation anymore because you've learned they don't matter.

If you're always the one compromising, that's not compromise. That's you abandoning yourself to keep the peace.

When Your Partner Makes You Choose

Some partners, consciously or unconsciously, make you choose between them and your life.

'It's your friends or me.' 'You spend too much time on your hobbies.' 'If you loved me, you'd want to spend all your time with me.' 'Your family is too demanding.'

This is manipulation. This is isolation. This is control disguised as love.

A healthy partner doesn't make you choose between them and your life. A healthy partner becomes part of your life while encouraging you to maintain all the other parts.

If your partner is threatened by:

- Your friendships

- Your family relationships
- Your hobbies
- Your career
- Your independence
- Your alone time

That's not love. That's possessiveness. And possessiveness isn't romantic. It's dangerous.

The Co-dependency Trap

Co-dependency feels like love. It feels like deep connection. It feels like you can't live without each other.

But it's not healthy intimacy. It's enmeshment. It's two people who can't function independently, who've merged their identities, who've become so tangled up that there's no clear boundary between them.

Signs of co-dependency:

- You can't make decisions without them
- You feel responsible for their emotions
- Their mood determines your mood
- You feel anxious when you're apart
- You've given up everything that made you yourself
- You enable their unhealthy behaviours because you can't stand conflict
- You're more focused on their needs than your own
- You feel like you'd be nothing without them

Co-dependency isn't romantic. It's a dysfunction that masquerades as devotion. And it will destroy both of you.

Real love is interdependent: two whole people who choose to share their lives. Co-dependency is two half-people clinging to each other to feel whole. One is healthy. The other is toxic.

Setting Boundaries in Romantic Relationships

You need boundaries in romantic relationships. Not because you don't love them. Because you do love them and you want the relationship to be sustainable.

Healthy relationship boundaries include:

- Time for yourself and your individual pursuits
- Maintaining friendships and family relationships
- Financial independence or clear financial boundaries
- Emotional independence (not responsible for their feelings)
- Physical boundaries (bodily autonomy, consent)
- Privacy (you're entitled to some things that are just yours)
- Limits on acceptable behaviour (no yelling, no name-calling, no manipulation)

Setting these boundaries doesn't mean you don't love them. It means you love yourself too. And sustainable love requires both.

When They Call You Selfish

When you start maintaining your identity, setting boundaries, and refusing to abandon yourself, your partner might call you selfish.

'You've changed.' 'You're not the person I fell in love with.' 'Why are you being so selfish?' 'Don't you love me anymore?'

This is manipulation. They're trying to guilt you back into self-abandonment.

Your response: 'I'm the same person. I'm just not abandoning myself anymore. If you fell in love with someone who had no boundaries and no identity, that wasn't the real me. That was me performing.'

A partner who loved the version of you that had no self won't like the version of you that does. And that tells you everything you need to know about whether they loved you or loved having someone to control.

The Different Love Languages of Self-Abandonment

Self-abandonment shows up differently for different people:

The Chameleon: You become whoever they need. You have no consistent identity because you're always adjusting to match them.

The Martyr: You sacrifice constantly and keep score internally. You give and give and resent and resent, but never say anything because that would be 'selfish.'

The Fixer: You make their problems your problems. You're constantly trying to rescue them, fix them, improve them. Their life becomes your project.

The People-Pleaser: You say yes to everything. You never express needs. You make yourself as low-maintenance as possible. You pride yourself on being 'easy.'

The Validator: Your entire purpose is to make them feel good about themselves. You exist to praise, admire, support, validate. Your feelings are irrelevant.

Recognize your pattern. Understand how you disappear. Then consciously choose to stay present.

The Work of Staying Yourself

Loving without losing yourself is active work. It doesn't happen automatically. You have to consciously choose yourself, over and over, even when it's uncomfortable.

Practical ways to stay yourself:

- Schedule time for your individual interests and protect it
- Maintain friendships actively, not just when convenient
- Check in with yourself regularly: What do I want? What do I feel? What matters to me?
- Practice expressing your actual opinions, not just agreeable ones
- Say no sometimes, even when you could say yes
- Keep pursuing your goals and dreams
- Have your own money, your own space (even if metaphorical), your own life

This isn't selfish. This is self-preservation. And it's the only way to build a sustainable relationship.

When the Relationship Ends and You Don't Know Who You Are

If you've lost yourself in a relationship and it ends, you'll face a terrifying question: who am I without them?

You'll realize you don't know what you like anymore. You don't have friends because you abandoned them. You don't have hobbies because you gave them up. You don't have goals because theirs became yours.

This is the cost of self-abandonment. When the relationship ends, you're not just grieving the relationship. You're grieving yourself.

And you have to rebuild from scratch. Rediscover who you are. Reconnect with old interests or find new ones. Repair friendships. Remember what you wanted before you forgot to want anything.

It's hard. It's lonely. It takes time.

But it's also an opportunity. An opportunity to build yourself back as a whole person this time. As someone who knows that love doesn't require self-erasure.

The Promise of Whole-Person Love

When you love someone without losing yourself, you get to experience what real love actually is:

Two whole people choosing each other. Not needing each other to feel complete. Not using each other to avoid themselves. Just... choosing. Every day. To share life. To support each other. To grow together while also growing individually.

That kind of love is sustainable. That kind of love doesn't burn out. That kind of love doesn't require one person to sacrifice their identity.

But you can't have that kind of love until you stop abandoning yourself. Until you believe that you are worthy of love as you actually are, not as some moulded version of what someone else needs.

So stay yourself. Keep your identity. Maintain your boundaries. Pursue your goals. Love fully, but don't lose yourself in the process.

You can have both. Love and selfhood. Partnership and identity. Connection and independence.

But only if you refuse to disappear.

Chapter 18: Boundaries Are Not Negotiable

Your partner wants to go through your phone. They want to know where you are every moment. They want access to your passwords. They want to isolate you from friends who 'don't support the relationship.' They want you available 24/7. They want to control what you wear, who you see, what you do.

And when you push back, they tell you that boundaries mean you don't trust them. That boundaries mean you're hiding something. That boundaries mean you don't really love them. That in a real relationship, there are no boundaries.

They're wrong.

Boundaries aren't optional in relationships. They're essential. And when someone tells you that boundaries are negotiable, they're telling you they plan to violate yours.

What Boundaries Actually Are

Boundaries in relationships are not walls. They're not about shutting your partner out. They're about maintaining healthy separation while building intimacy.

Boundaries are:

- Lines that define where you end and they begin
- Limits on what behaviour you'll accept
- Protection for your autonomy and personhood
- Guidelines for how you want to be treated

• Non-negotiable standards for the relationship

Healthy boundaries in romantic relationships include:

• Physical boundaries (consent, bodily autonomy)
• Emotional boundaries (not responsible for their feelings)
• Time boundaries (alone time, time with others)
• Privacy boundaries (some things can be private)
• Financial boundaries (money management)
• Communication boundaries (how you talk to each other)
• Behavioural boundaries (what treatment is acceptable)

These aren't optional. These aren't negotiable. These are the foundation of a healthy relationship.

The 'No Boundaries' Myth

There's this romantic idea that true love means no boundaries. That you should share everything, know everything, be completely merged with your partner. That privacy is suspicious. That independence is selfish. That boundaries mean you're not really in love.

This is toxic relationship propaganda.

Healthy relationships have boundaries. Clear ones. Respected ones. Non-negotiable ones.

You're allowed to:

• Have a password-protected phone
• Have conversations that are private
• Have relationships outside the romantic relationship
• Have time alone

- Have thoughts and feelings you don't share
- Have autonomy over your own body, time, and choices
- Say no to things you don't want to do

None of these mean you don't love them. They mean you're a separate person. Which you are. Even in a relationship.

Common Boundary Violations in Relationships

Let's name the violations so you can recognize them:

Checking your phone/email without permission: This is a violation. Your phone is private. Your communications are private. Access is not automatic just because you're in a relationship.

Demanding to know your whereabouts constantly: 'Where are you? Who are you with? When will you be home? What are you doing?' on repeat is surveillance, not love.

Isolating you from friends and family: 'I don't like your friends.' 'Your family is too demanding.' 'Choose me or them.' This is control, not closeness.

Controlling what you wear: Your body, your clothes. If they're policing your appearance, that's a boundary violation.

Demanding access to your money: Financial boundaries matter. You're entitled to financial independence or clear agreements about money.

Pushing past 'no' in any context: No is a complete sentence. If they keep pushing after you've said no, to sex, to plans, to anything, that's a violation.

Making you responsible for their emotions: If your job is to manage their feelings, prevent their anger, or maintain their happiness, that's a boundary violation. You're not their emotional support animal.

Punishing you for having boundaries: If they sulk, rage, give silent treatment, or withdraw affection when you set boundaries, that's manipulation.

When They Say Boundaries Mean You Don't Trust Them

This is manipulation. Let's break it down:

'If you loved me, you'd share your passwords.' No. If they loved you, they'd respect your privacy.

'If you trusted me, you wouldn't need boundaries.' No. Trust doesn't mean unlimited access. Trust means confidence that boundaries will be respected.

'Boundaries are for people who have something to hide.' No. Boundaries are for people who have a self to protect.

'In a real relationship, there are no secrets.' Having privacy isn't the same as keeping secrets. You're entitled to thoughts, conversations, and experiences that are just yours.

Your response to any of these: 'Boundaries are healthy. They're non-negotiable. If you can't respect them, we can't continue.'

Don't argue. Don't justify. Don't explain why you deserve privacy. You just do. It's not up for debate.

The Different Flavors of Boundary Violation

The Slow Erosion: They don't violate all your boundaries at once. They test one. Then another. Each violation is small, so you feel like maybe you're overreacting. But slowly, all your boundaries disappear.

This is intentional. It's easier to boil a frog slowly. If they violated all your boundaries at once, you'd leave. So they do it incrementally.

The Emotional Blackmail: 'If you don't [violate your boundary], then I'll [consequence].' 'If you go out with your friends, I'll be so hurt.' 'If you don't share your password, I'll know you're cheating.'

This is manipulation. Your boundaries shouldn't require you to manage their emotional reactions.

The Gaslighting: 'I never said that.' 'You're overreacting.' 'You're too sensitive.' 'That didn't happen the way you remember.' They violate your boundaries then make you question whether it even happened.

Trust yourself. If it feels like a violation, it is.

The Rationalization: 'I only checked your phone because I love you.' 'I only ask where you are because I worry.' 'I only want to spend all our time together because you're important to me.'

Love doesn't justify boundary violations. Worry doesn't justify surveillance. Importance doesn't justify control.

Setting Boundaries With Someone Who Doesn't Want Them

Here's the hard truth: you can't make someone respect your boundaries. You can only enforce consequences when they don't.

Steps for setting boundaries in a relationship:

1. Be clear: 'I need privacy. I won't be sharing my phone password. This isn't negotiable.'

Direct. Specific. Non-negotiable. No room for interpretation.

2. State the consequence: 'If you go through my phone without permission, that's a serious violation of trust and we'll need to seriously reconsider this relationship.'

They need to know what happens if they violate the boundary.

3. Follow through: This is the hard part. When they violate the boundary, and if they don't respect boundaries, they will, you enforce the consequence.

If you said you'd reconsider the relationship, reconsider it. If you said you'd leave, leave. If you said you'd take space, take space.

Boundaries without enforcement are suggestions. And suggestions get ignored.

4. Don't negotiate: When they push back, and they will, don't engage in a debate about whether your boundary is reasonable. It's yours. It's non-negotiable.

'This is my boundary. I'm not debating it.'

5. Be prepared to walk away: If they can't respect your boundaries, the relationship can't continue. Be ready to end it if necessary.

This is the ultimate enforcement. And sometimes it's the only thing that works.

The Cycle of Boundary Violation

In unhealthy relationships, boundary violations follow a predictable pattern:

1. They violate a boundary

2. You get upset

3. They apologize, promise it won't happen again, make you feel like you're overreacting

4. You forgive them

5. Things are good for a while

6. They violate the boundary again, or a different one

7. Repeat

Each cycle, they push a little further. Each cycle, your boundaries get weaker. Each cycle, you're more worn down.

Breaking this cycle requires:

- Recognizing the pattern
- Stopping the cycle at step 4 (don't forgive without changed behaviour)
- Enforcing real consequences

• Being willing to leave if the pattern continues

Apologies without changed behaviour are manipulation. Don't fall for them.

What Healthy Boundary Respect Looks Like

In healthy relationships, boundaries are respected. Here's what that looks like:

• You state a boundary once and it's honoured

• They don't push back, negotiate, or make you feel bad for having it

• They might not understand the boundary, but they respect it anyway

• They remember your boundaries and don't repeatedly 'forget'

• They have boundaries too, and you respect each other's

• Boundaries are seen as healthy parts of the relationship, not threats to it

If your partner consistently respects your boundaries, even when they don't fully understand them, that's green flag behaviour.

If your partner consistently violates, dismisses, or argues with your boundaries, that's a red flag. A big one.

Financial Boundaries

Let's talk specifically about money because this trips people up:

You're entitled to financial boundaries even in serious relationships:

- Your own bank account
- Your own credit cards
- Your own financial decisions about your money
- Your own savings
- Privacy about your finances if you choose

'But we're partners, we should share everything!' No. Financial enmeshment is dangerous. You should have some level of financial independence.

Even if you share finances, you can have boundaries:

- Amounts you can spend without consulting each other
- Individual discretionary money
- Financial transparency without giving up all autonomy

Financial abuse often starts with erosion of financial boundaries. Protect yours.

Physical and Sexual Boundaries

Your body is yours. Always. In all contexts. Including in a relationship.

You are allowed to:

- Say no to sex, any time, for any reason
- Have preferences about sexual activities
- Need time before being ready for physical intimacy
- Change your mind about what you're comfortable with
- Have bodily autonomy

Consent is ongoing. It's enthusiastic. It can be withdrawn at any point. And it's required every single time.

If your partner:

- Pressures you for sex
- Guilts you when you say no
- Pushes past boundaries you've stated
- Makes you feel obligated to have sex
- Doesn't respect your no

That's abuse. Full stop. Leave.

The 'Crazy' Label

When you start setting and enforcing boundaries, you might be called crazy. Controlling. Paranoid. Difficult. Too much.

This is a tactic. It's designed to make you doubt yourself and your boundaries.

You're not crazy for:

- Wanting privacy
- Needing alone time
- Maintaining friendships
- Having standards for how you're treated
- Enforcing consequences for violations
- Leaving when boundaries aren't respected

If someone calls you crazy for having reasonable boundaries, they're showing you who they are. Believe them.

When to Leave

Leave when:

- They consistently violate your boundaries
- They punish you for having boundaries
- They escalate violations despite consequences
- They make you feel crazy for having normal boundaries
- They isolate you from everyone who might support your boundaries
- You feel unsafe
- Your boundaries are seen as threats rather than healthy limits

Don't wait for it to get better. If they don't respect boundaries early, they won't respect them later. The pattern is established.

Leaving isn't giving up. Leaving is recognizing that you deserve a partner who respects you. And respect includes respecting boundaries.

Your Non-Negotiables

Before you get into a relationship, or right now if you're already in one, get clear on your non-negotiables:

What boundaries will you not compromise on?

- Privacy boundaries?
- Time boundaries?
- Friendship boundaries?
- Physical boundaries?

- Communication boundaries?
- Financial boundaries?

Write them down. Be clear about them. And when someone violates them, enforce consequences immediately.

Your boundaries are not negotiable. Not for love. Not for companionship. Not because you're afraid of being alone. Not ever.

Boundaries are the foundation of healthy relationships. Without them, you don't have partnership. You have enmeshment, control, or abuse.

So set them. State them clearly. Enforce them consistently. And leave relationships that don't respect them.

Boundaries are not negotiable.

Chapter 19: Red Flags and Green Flags

You know that feeling when something's off, but you can't quite name it? When you're trying to convince yourself that this person is great even though your gut is screaming at you to run? When you're making excuses for behaviour, you'd never accept from anyone else?

That's your nervous system trying to tell you something.

This chapter is about learning to recognize red flags early, before you're too invested to see clearly. And equally important: learning to recognize green flags so you know what healthy actually looks like.

Why We Miss Red Flags

You miss red flags because:

You're looking for the best in people: This is admirable. It's also dangerous. Not everyone deserves the benefit of the doubt. Some people show you exactly who they are early. Believe them.

You think love can fix it: If you just love them enough, they'll change. If you're patient enough, understanding enough, supportive enough, they'll become the person you need them to be. They won't.

You're afraid of being alone: A bad relationship feels better than no relationship. It doesn't. But the fear convinces you to ignore what you're seeing.

You're attracted to what's familiar: If you grew up with dysfunction, dysfunction feels like home. The red flags feel comfortable because they match your childhood. That doesn't make them acceptable.

You rationalize: 'Everyone has flaws.' 'I'm not perfect either.' 'It's not that bad.' 'They're just going through a hard time.' Stop. Red flags are red flags, not personality quirks.

Your job isn't to give everyone infinite chances. Your job is to protect yourself by paying attention to warning signs.

The Early Red Flags

These are the red flags that show up early. Pay attention. Act on them. Don't wait to see if they 'get better.'

Love bombing: They're too into you too fast. Overwhelming attention, grand gestures, intense declarations of love, talking about the future immediately. This isn't romance. It's a manipulation tactic.

Real connection builds over time. Instant intensity is a warning sign, not a fairy tale.

Disrespecting your boundaries early: 'I know you said you need to go, but just stay a little longer.' 'I know you said you're not ready for that, but...' They're showing you they don't respect your no. Believe them.

If they don't respect small boundaries early, they won't respect big ones later.

Rushing intimacy: Pushing for physical intimacy before you're ready. Pushing for emotional intimacy (oversharing, demanding you overshare) too fast. Pushing for commitment too soon.

This isn't passion. This is someone trying to lock you in before you see who they really are.

Bad-mouthing all their exes: If everyone they've ever dated is 'crazy,' the common denominator is them. One bad relationship? Okay. Every relationship? They're the problem.

Jekyll and Hyde behaviour: They're amazing sometimes and terrible others. Sweet then mean. Attentive then neglectful. The inconsistency is the red flag.

You can't fix inconsistency by being better. It's not about you. It's about them.

Isolating you early: They want all your time. They're jealous of your friends. They don't like when you have plans without them. This is control, not devotion.

Making you responsible for their emotions: 'If you leave, I'll be devastated.' 'You're the only thing keeping me sane.' 'If you loved me, you'd...' This is emotional manipulation.

You're not responsible for their emotional regulation. You're not their therapist or their saviour.

The Mid-Relationship Red Flags

These red flags appear after you're already invested. They're harder to see because you're attached. They're not harder to act on. You just have more to lose.

Gaslighting: 'That didn't happen.' 'You're remembering wrong.' 'You're too sensitive.' 'I never said that.' They make you doubt your reality, your memory, your perceptions.

This is abuse. Full stop.

Financial control: They control the money. They monitor your spending. They make you ask for money. They sabotage your career. They create financial dependence.

Financial abuse is real abuse. It traps you.

Escalating violations: Boundaries you set keep getting violated. 'Apologies' are followed by the same behaviour. Each violation is a little worse than the last.

This pattern doesn't reverse. It escalates.

Punishing your independence: When you spend time with friends, they sulk. When you pursue your interests, they're hurt. When you need alone time, they make you feel guilty.

They want you dependent. That's not love.

Walking on eggshells: You're constantly monitoring their mood. Adjusting your behaviour to prevent their anger. Never sure what will set them off.

This is not a partnership. This is you managing an unstable person.

Double standards: Rules apply to you but not to them. They can have friends of the opposite sex, but you can't. They can have privacy, but you can't. They can make plans, but you need permission.

Hypocrisy is a red flag.

The Serious Red Flags

These are the flags that mean leave now. Not later. Not after one more chance. Now.

Any physical violence: Shoving, grabbing, hitting, throwing things at you. One time is too many times. Don't wait for it to escalate.

Threats: Threats to hurt you, hurt themselves, hurt people you love, ruin your life, take your kids. Any threat is serious.

Stalking behaviour: Showing up unannounced. Tracking your phone. Following you. Monitoring your online activity obsessively.

Forced sexual activity: Coercion, pressure, forcing, any sex without enthusiastic ongoing consent.

Complete isolation: They've successfully isolated you from friends, family, support systems. You have no one but them.

If any of these are happening, this is abuse. You need to leave safely. Contact domestic violence resources. Make a safety plan. Get help.

How to Spot Red Flags Early

Pay attention to:

How they treat service workers: Rude to waiters, baristas, retail workers? They'll eventually be rude to you. How people treat those with less power reveals character.

How they talk about others: Constantly criticizing, judging, gossiping? That's how they'll talk about you eventually.

How they handle disagreement: Do they listen? Respect your perspective? Or do they need to be right? Dismiss your views? Get defensive?

How they handle your boundaries: Do they respect them immediately? Or push, test, negotiate? Early boundary respect predicts later behaviour.

How they talk about their ex: With respect even though it didn't work out? Or with contempt, blame, and 'crazy' labels?

Whether they take accountability: Do they own their mistakes? Apologize genuinely? Or blame others, make excuses, deflect?

How you feel around them: Energized or drained? Safe or anxious? Yourself or performing? Your body knows things your mind rationalizes away.

Trust your gut. If something feels off, it probably is.

Green Flags (What Healthy Actually Looks Like)

Now let's talk about what to look for. What healthy looks like. Because if you grew up with dysfunction, you might not recognize healthy when you see it.

They respect your no: The first time. Without pushing. Without pouting. Without negotiating. 'No' is enough.

They're consistent: Who they are on date three is who they are on date thirty. No Jekyll and Hyde. No 'best behaviour' followed by real behaviour.

They encourage your independence: They support your friendships, your hobbies, your career, your goals. They're not threatened by you having a life outside them.

They take accountability: They apologize genuinely when they mess up. They don't make excuses. They change behaviour.

They communicate clearly: They tell you what they want, what they feel, what they need. They don't make you guess. They don't use mind games.

They respect your pace: They don't rush you into anything. Physical intimacy, emotional intimacy, commitment. They let things develop naturally.

They have healthy relationships: With friends, family, exes (or at least speak respectfully about exes). People who maintain healthy relationships can have healthy relationships.

They're emotionally regulated: They have feelings like everyone else, but they manage them. They don't expect you to regulate their emotions.

They're proud of you: They celebrate your wins. They support your growth. They want you to succeed, even in areas that have nothing to do with them.

You feel like yourself: You don't have to perform. You can be authentic. You feel more yourself with them, not less.

Yellow Flags (Proceed With Caution)

Not everything is a dealbreaker. Some things are yellow flags. Things to watch, to discuss, to see if they improve.

Poor communication skills: They struggle to express feelings or needs. This can improve if they're willing to work on it.

Emotional unavailability: They have walls up. This might be trauma. It might improve. Or it might be who they are. Give it limited time to see.

Different conflict styles: They avoid conflict while you address it, or vice versa. This can be worked through with effort from both people.

Recent major loss: They're grieving, processing trauma, going through something hard. They might not be emotionally available for a relationship right now. That's okay, but know what you're getting into.

Lifestyle incompatibilities: Different ideas about money, future plans, family. These aren't inherently red flags, but they need to be discussed early.

Yellow flags become red flags if:

- They refuse to work on the issue
- They blame you for the issue
- The pattern continues despite discussion
- They get defensive when you bring it up

Give yellow flags limited time and attention. If they don't improve, they become red.

The Pattern Recognition Exercise

Look at your relationship history. Are there patterns?

• Do you keep dating the same person in different bodies?

• Do the same red flags keep appearing?

• Do your relationships follow similar trajectories?

• Are you attracted to similar types who all have similar problems?

If yes, that's your nervous system seeking what's familiar. And if what's familiar is dysfunction, you're unconsciously choosing dysfunction.

Break the pattern by:

• Recognizing what you're attracted to and why

• Understanding what feels 'exciting' versus what's actually healthy

• Choosing differently even when it feels boring or uncomfortable

• Dating people who feel unfamiliar in good ways

Healthy might feel boring at first if you're used to drama. That's okay. Boring is good. Boring is stable. Boring is safe.

When Friends Point Out Red Flags

'I don't like how they talk to you.' 'This doesn't seem healthy.' 'I'm worried about you.' 'They remind me of your ex.'

Listen.

Your friends can see what you can't when you're emotionally invested. They're not jealous. They're not trying to ruin your happiness. They're seeing red flags you're rationalizing away.

If multiple trusted people are expressing concern, pay attention. You don't have to leave immediately. But you do need to seriously consider what they're seeing.

The Red Flag Checklist

Use this as a quick reference. If you can check off several items, you need to seriously reconsider the relationship.

Red flags:

- Love bombing/moving too fast
- Boundary violations
- Bad-mouths all exes
- Wants all your time/isolates you
- Makes you responsible for their emotions
- Gaslighting
- Financial control
- Punishes your independence
- You're walking on eggshells
- Double standards
- Any violence or threats
- You feel worse about yourself
- You're constantly anxious
- Your friends/family are concerned
- You're making excuses for their behaviour

Green flags:

- Respects your boundaries
- Consistent behaviour
- Encourages your independence
- Takes accountability
- Communicates clearly
- Respects your pace
- Has healthy relationships
- Emotionally regulated
- Proud of you
- You feel like yourself
- You feel safe
- You feel respected
- Conflicts are productive
- They support your growth
- Your friends/family like them

What to Do When You See Red Flags

Early red flags (first few dates/months): End it. You're not invested yet. Trust your gut. There are other people out there without these flags.

Mid-relationship red flags: Address them directly. 'This behaviour isn't acceptable. It needs to change.' Give them one chance to change. Watch for actual changed behaviour, not just apologies.

Serious red flags: Leave. Make a safety plan if needed. Get support. Don't give more chances.

Remember: You're not obligated to give infinite chances. You're not obligated to stay because you've invested time. You're not obligated to fix someone who shows you they're not safe. Red flags are information. Use it. Green flags are what you deserve. Wait for them.

PART SIX
THE PRACTICE

Chapter 20: The 30-Day Emotional Hygiene Reset

You've read the whole book. You understand the concepts. You see the patterns. You recognize your family dynamics in your friendships, your parent-boss confusion, your tendency to lose yourself in relationships, your inability to set boundaries.

Now what?

Knowledge is useless without practice. Understanding your patterns doesn't change them. You have to actively work to build new habits, new responses, new ways of being.

This chapter is your 30-day reset. A practical, day-by-day guide to implementing emotional hygiene. Not because 30 days will fix everything. It won't. But because 30 days is enough time to start building new patterns and see real change.

Before You Start

Set yourself up for success:

Get a journal: Digital or physical, doesn't matter. You need somewhere to track your progress, note your observations, work through your thoughts.

Choose your focus area: You can't tackle everything at once. Pick the area that's causing you the most pain right now. Family boundaries? Workplace dynamics? Romantic relationship? Friendships? Start there.

Tell someone: Accountability helps. Tell a trusted friend what you're doing. Check in with them weekly. Or find an online community. Don't do this entirely alone.

Lower your expectations: You will not be perfect. You will slip. You will backslide. That's normal. Progress, not perfection.

Schedule the time: These practices take time. Block it in your calendar like any other important appointment.

Week One: Awareness and Assessment

You can't change what you don't see. Week one is about building awareness of your current patterns.

Day 1: Identify Your Patterns

Journal prompt: What are the three most persistent patterns in my relationships? (Examples: I always say yes even when I want to say no. I take on other people's problems. I disappear into relationships. I seek approval from authority figures.)

Be specific. Be honest. No judgment, just observation.

Day 2: Trace the Origin

For each pattern you identified, ask: Where did I learn this? What message did I internalize that created this pattern?

Understanding the origin doesn't excuse the behaviour, but it helps you see why it's so ingrained.

Day 3: Assess the Cost

For each pattern, write: What is this pattern costing me? (Time, energy, relationships, self-respect, mental health, opportunities)

Get clear on what you're sacrificing by maintaining these patterns.

Day 4: Name Your Boundaries

List your non-negotiable boundaries. What treatment will you no longer accept? What behaviours will you no longer tolerate? What will you no longer do out of guilt or obligation?

Be specific. 'Better boundaries' is vague. 'I will not answer work emails after 7pm' is specific.

Day 5: The Relationship Audit

List your significant relationships (family, friends, romantic, work). For each, rate it 1-10 on: Do I feel energized or drained? Can I be myself? Is it reciprocal? Do they respect my boundaries?

This shows you where the problems are concentrated.

Day 6: Identify Your Triggers

What situations consistently trigger your old patterns? (Examples: When my mother calls. When my boss asks for something. When I'm dating someone new. When a friend needs help.)

Knowing your triggers helps you prepare better responses.

Day 7: Weekly Review

Review what you learned this week. What surprised you? What was hard to acknowledge? What pattern do you most want to change? Write it down.

Week Two: Building Boundaries

Now that you see the patterns, start interrupting them with boundaries.

Day 8: The Easy No

Practice saying no to something small and low-stakes. 'No thanks' to something you don't want. Don't explain. Don't apologize. Just practice the no.

Build the muscle with easy reps first.

Day 9: The Medium No

Say no to something that triggers mild guilt. Decline an invitation. Turn down a request for help. Set a small boundary.

Notice the guilt. Feel it. Don't act on it. The boundary stands.

Day 10: Stop Explaining

Today, when you say no to anything, don't explain why. Just 'No, thank you' or 'That doesn't work for me.'

Notice how uncomfortable this is. Notice the urge to justify. Resist it.

Day 11: Set a Time Boundary

Pick one time boundary and enforce it today. Leave work on time. Don't check email after a certain hour. Take your full lunch break. Something.

Practice protecting your time like it matters. Because it does.

Day 12: Address a Violation

Someone violated a boundary (or will today. They usually do). Address it immediately. 'I need you to stop doing X.' 'That's not okay with me.' 'I said no.'

Don't let it slide. Enforce in the moment.

Day 13: Let Someone Be Disappointed

Today, let someone be disappointed in you without trying to fix it. They're upset you set a boundary? Let them be upset. You're not managing their feelings.

This is hard. Do it anyway.

Day 14: Weekly Review

How did boundary-setting go? What was hardest? What got easier? Did you cave on anything? What did you learn? Write it down.

Week Three: Changing Relationship Dynamics

Boundaries are set. Now start changing how you show up in relationships.

Day 15: Stop Rescuing

Someone has a crisis that's not yours. Don't rescue them. Ask 'What's your plan for handling this?' instead of offering to fix it.

Let them solve their own problems. You're not responsible for everyone.

Day 16: Stop People-Pleasing

Express an opinion that's actually yours, even if it differs from the group. State a preference. Make a choice based on what you want, not what will make others happy.

Practice being yourself, not a mirror.

Day 17: Ask for What You Need

Identify something you need (help, support, time, something specific). Ask for it directly. No hinting. No hoping they'll notice. Ask.

Your needs are valid. Practice stating them.

Day 18: Stop Over-Functioning

In one relationship where you typically do too much, do less. Let someone else handle it. Let the ball drop if necessary.

You're not responsible for everything. Stop acting like you are.

Day 19: Disagree Out Loud

When you disagree with something, say so. Don't just go along. Don't smooth it over. State your different perspective.

Conflict isn't catastrophic. Practice tolerating it.

Day 20: Reclaim Your Time

Do something just for you today. Not productive. Not for anyone else. Just because you enjoy it. Protect this time fiercely.

Your joy matters. Act like it.

Day 21: Weekly Review

How did relationship dynamics shift? What was uncomfortable? What felt good? What resistance did you encounter? From others? From yourself? Write it down.

Week Four: Integration and Commitment

Final week. Solidify the changes. Commit to continuing.

Day 22: Have a Hard Conversation

Address something you've been avoiding. Set a boundary you've been too scared to set. Have the conversation you've been putting off.

Scared is okay. Do it scared.

Day 23: Enforce a Consequence

Someone violated a boundary you set. Enforce the consequence you stated. Actually do what you said you'd do.

Boundaries without enforcement are suggestions. Enforce.

Day 24: Assess Progress

Compare today to day one. What's different? What's easier? What still feels impossible? What surprised you? Be honest about progress and areas still needing work.

Day 25: Identify Your Supporters

Who in your life supports these changes? Who respects your boundaries? Who encourages your growth? Invest more in those relationships.

Also identify who pushes back. Create distance there.

Day 26: Plan for Maintenance

What practices will you continue after these 30 days? Daily check-ins? Weekly boundary assessment? Monthly relationship audit? Schedule them.

This isn't a one-time thing. It's ongoing.

Day 27: Write Your Non-Negotiables

Based on what you learned, write your updated list of non-negotiables. What will you absolutely not tolerate going forward? What boundaries are permanent?

This is your line in the sand. Know it. Defend it.

Day 28: Celebrate Progress

Acknowledge what you've accomplished. You've been doing hard work. You've been changing lifelong patterns. That deserves recognition.

Write down your wins. All of them. Big and small.

Day 29: Anticipate Challenges

What situations will test these new patterns? (Holidays with family? Conflict at work? Dating someone new?) Plan for them. What will you do differently?

Preparation helps. Think ahead.

Day 30: Commitment

Write a commitment to yourself. What are you committing to continuing? What boundaries are permanent? What person are you becoming?

This is a contract with yourself. Take it seriously.

The Daily Practices

Beyond the daily assignments, integrate these ongoing practices:

Morning Check-In (2 minutes):

Each morning, ask yourself: What's one boundary I need to hold today? What's one old pattern I want to interrupt? How do I want to show up today?

Evening Audit (5 minutes):

Each evening, reflect: Did I honour my boundaries? Where did I slip? What triggered my old patterns? What did I do well? What will I do differently tomorrow?

Weekly Reset (15 minutes):

Each week, do a bigger review: What patterns am I noticing? What boundaries need reinforcing? What relationships need attention? What's working? What isn't?

Tracking Your Progress

Use your journal to track:

- Boundaries set and enforced
- Times you said no without apologizing
- Moments you chose yourself over people-pleasing
- Instances of asking for what you need
- Relationships that improved or got worse
- Feelings that came up
- Old patterns you successfully interrupted
- New patterns you're building

This data shows you your progress. Some days you won't feel like you're getting anywhere. The data will prove otherwise.

What to Expect

During these 30 days, you'll likely experience:

Discomfort: Changing lifelong patterns is uncomfortable. You'll feel guilty, anxious, scared. That's normal. Discomfort is not damage.

Pushback: People who benefited from your lack of boundaries will push back. They'll test your boundaries. They'll make you feel bad. Hold firm.

Relief: As you start honouring yourself, you'll feel lighter. More yourself. Less burdened by everyone else's stuff.

Loneliness: Some relationships will change or end. You might feel lonely before you find your people. That's temporary.

Clarity: You'll get clearer on who you are, what you want, what you'll accept. This clarity is powerful.

Setbacks: You will backslide. You will fall into old patterns. That's not failure. That's part of the process.

After the 30 Days

This isn't over at day 30. This is the beginning.

Keep going with:

- Daily check-ins and evening audits
- Weekly reviews and adjustments
- Monthly deep dives into relationship dynamics
- Ongoing boundary setting and enforcement
- Continued work on the patterns

Emotional hygiene is not a one-time fix. It's a practice. Like brushing your teeth. You don't do it once and declare yourself done. You do it every day, consistently, because it matters.

Some days will be easier than others. Some days you'll feel like you've mastered this. Some days you'll feel like you've learned nothing. Both are normal.

Keep going.

The Real Goal

The goal isn't perfection. The goal isn't to never slip, never struggle, never fall back into old patterns.

The goal is awareness. The goal is catching yourself faster. The goal is choosing yourself more often than you abandon yourself. The goal is building a life where your boundaries are respected, your needs matter, and you're not constantly sacrificing yourself for everyone else.

The goal is freedom. Freedom from the exhausting burden of people-pleasing. Freedom from the constant anxiety of seeking approval. Freedom from relationships that drain you. Freedom to be yourself without apology.

That's worth 30 days. That's worth a lifetime of practice.

So start. Day one is tomorrow. Or today. Or right now.

Start.

Chapter 21: When You Slip (Because You Will)

You will slip. Let's just establish that right now. You will fall back into old patterns. You will say yes when you meant to say no. You will abandon a boundary you swore you'd hold. You will people-please after swearing you were done. You will disappear into a relationship again. You will seek approval you said you didn't need.

This is not failure. This is part of the process.

This chapter is about what to do when you slip. Not if. When. Because you're human, and humans don't change in straight lines. We change in spirals, in stops and starts, with progress and setbacks.

Why You'll Slip

You'll slip because:

Old patterns are deeply wired: You've been running these patterns for years, maybe decades. Your nervous system defaults to what's familiar. Changing that takes time and consistent practice. You will default to the old pattern sometimes.

Stress triggers regression: When you're stressed, tired, overwhelmed, your brain goes into survival mode. And survival mode uses the oldest, most established patterns. The ones you're trying to change.

Some people are better at pushing your buttons: Your family knows exactly how to trigger you. That person at work who reminds you of your critical parent. That romantic partner who makes you feel like you're never enough. They'll find the weak spots in your new boundaries.

You'll forget: In the moment, you'll forget all your new tools. You'll forget that you were supposed to say no. You'll forget that you don't have to fix everyone's problems. You'll forget that their emergency isn't yours.

You'll rationalize: 'Just this once.' 'It's a special circumstance.' 'I don't want to be difficult.' The rationalizations are sneaky. And sometimes convincing.

Change is hard: Really hard. And sometimes you'll get tired of doing the hard thing. You'll want to go back to what's easy, even when easy is harmful.

All of this is normal. Expected. Part of the process.

What Slipping Looks Like

You might not even realize you've slipped immediately. Here's what it looks like:

- You agreed to something you didn't want to do
- You worked late/through lunch/on your day off when you said you wouldn't
- You let a boundary violation slide without addressing it
- You took on someone else's problem as your own
- You moulded yourself to fit what someone else wanted
- You said yes when you meant no
- You avoided a hard conversation you needed to have
- You sought approval you said you didn't need
- You made yourself small to keep the peace

• You abandoned yourself to maintain a relationship

Sometimes you'll realize immediately. 'Oh no, I just did the thing I said I wouldn't do.' Sometimes you won't realize until later. 'Wait, when did I agree to that?'

Either way, the realization feels bad. Disappointing. Like you've failed. Like all your work was for nothing.

It wasn't. You didn't fail. You're learning. And learning includes mistakes.

What Not to Do When You Slip

Don't spiral into shame: 'I'm so stupid. I'll never change. I'm broken. What's wrong with me?' Stop. Shame doesn't help. Shame makes it worse. Shame makes you more likely to keep slipping because you feel hopeless.

One slip doesn't erase all your progress. You're not back at square one. You just stumbled. That's different from falling.

Don't give up: 'I slipped once so I might as well keep slipping. I clearly can't do this. Why bother trying?' No. One slip doesn't mean throw away all your boundaries and go back to your old patterns.

You don't abandon your entire diet because you ate one cookie. Same principle.

Don't double down on the slip: 'Well, I already said yes to this thing I didn't want to do, so I might as well also say yes to this other thing.' No. Stop the pattern as soon as you notice it.

One slip doesn't give you permission to slip all day/week/month. Course correct immediately.

Don't ignore it: Pretending it didn't happen doesn't help. You did slip. Acknowledge it. Learn from it. Move forward.

What to Do When You Slip

1. Notice it: The first step is awareness. You slipped. You fell into an old pattern. Name it. 'I just said yes when I wanted to say no.' 'I just took on their problem.' 'I just abandoned my boundary.'

Noticing is progress. A year ago you might not have even realized you slipped.

2. Understand why: What triggered the slip? Stress? A specific person? Fatigue? Fear? Understanding the trigger helps you prepare better next time.

'I slipped because my mother called and I regressed to people-pleasing child mode.' That's useful information.

3. Self-compassion: Talk to yourself the way you'd talk to a friend. 'This is hard. I'm learning. I made a mistake. That's okay. I'm not perfect and I don't need to be.'

Be kind to yourself. You're doing something difficult. You deserve compassion, not criticism.

4. Course correct if possible: Can you undo the slip? Can you go back and say 'Actually, I need to change my answer to no'? Can you address the boundary violation you let slide?

It's not always possible. But sometimes it is. If you can course correct, do it.

5. Learn from it: What would you do differently next time? What can you prepare for? What boundary needs reinforcing?

Every slip is data. Use it.

6. Get back on track: One slip doesn't define you. Get back to your boundaries. Get back to honouring yourself. Get back to the work.

Don't wallow. Just resume the practice.

The Different Types of Slips

The Autopilot Slip: You slipped because you weren't paying attention. Someone asked and you said yes before thinking. This happens when the pattern is deeply automatic.

Fix: Pause before answering. 'Let me think about that and get back to you.' Give yourself time to check in with what you actually want.

The Pressure Slip: You slipped because someone pushed hard and you caved. The guilt, the manipulation, the pressure was too much in the moment.

Fix: Practice holding your boundary under pressure. Expect pressure. Prepare responses. 'I understand you're disappointed. My answer is still no.'

The Exhaustion Slip: You slipped because you were too tired to hold the boundary. Saying no takes energy. Sometimes you don't have it.

Fix: Protect your energy better. Rest more. Say no to smaller things so you have energy for the bigger boundaries.

The Fear Slip: You slipped because you were scared. Scared of conflict. Scared of disappointing them. Scared of being alone. Scared of consequences.

Fix: Work on tolerating the fear. Feel it and hold the boundary anyway. The fear doesn't have to dictate your choices.

The Rationalization Slip: You slipped because you convinced yourself this was different. A special case. An exception. 'Just this once.'

Fix: Watch for rationalization. When you start telling yourself why this time is different, that's a red flag. Boundaries don't have exceptions just because it's easier to cave.

The Difference Between a Slip and a Pattern

One slip is a mistake. A pattern of slips is a problem.

A slip: You held your boundaries for weeks. Then one day, under pressure, you caved. You notice. You feel bad. You course correct. You get back on track.

A pattern: You keep slipping with the same person, in the same situations, using the same rationalizations. You notice but don't change anything. The slips become frequent. You're barely holding boundaries at all anymore.

If you're slipping repeatedly, you need to:

• Identify the specific trigger or person causing the pattern

• Strengthen that specific boundary

• Get additional support (therapy, accountability partner, etc.)

• Consider whether you need distance from the person/situation

Occasional slips are normal. Constant slips mean something needs to change.

When Slipping Becomes a Cycle

Sometimes slipping becomes a cycle:

1. You set a boundary

2. You hold it for a while

3. You slip

4. You feel guilty/ashamed

5. You recommit to the boundary

6. You hold it for a while

7. You slip again

8. Repeat

If you're in this cycle, you're not hopeless. But you need to interrupt it:

Change your environment: If a specific person or situation keeps triggering slips, you might need distance.

You can't hold boundaries around people who constantly assault them if you're in constant contact.

Get support: You might need help. A therapist. A support group. An accountability partner. Someone who can help you see the pattern and interrupt it.

Strengthen the boundary: Maybe the boundary isn't clear enough. Make it more specific. Make the consequences more immediate. Make it harder to slip.

Address the underlying issue: Why do you keep slipping? What fear or need is driving this? Maybe you need to work on that specifically.

The Shame Spiral

The most dangerous part of slipping isn't the slip itself. It's the shame spiral that can follow.

Slip → Shame → 'I'm a failure' → Give up on all boundaries → Slip more → More shame → Full regression to old patterns.

Break this spiral with self-compassion:

- 'I slipped. That's okay. I'm human.'
- 'This doesn't erase my progress.'
- 'I can get back on track right now.'
- 'I'm learning. Learning includes mistakes.'
- 'One slip doesn't define me.'

Shame makes everything worse. Compassion makes recovery possible.

Using Slips as Information

Every slip tells you something:

- Which boundaries are hardest to hold?
- Which people or situations trigger your old patterns?
- What fears are still running the show?
- What additional support you need?
- Where you need to strengthen your practice?

Track your slips. Look for patterns. Use the information to get better at this.

Slips aren't failures. They're feedback.

The Long Game

You're playing the long game here. This isn't about perfect execution. It's about overall trajectory.

Are you slipping less than you were six months ago? Are you noticing faster? Are you course correcting quicker? Are you holding boundaries more often than you're abandoning them?

If yes, you're winning. Even if you slipped yesterday. Even if you'll slip tomorrow.

Progress isn't linear. It's messy. It includes setbacks. But if the overall trend is toward healthier boundaries, more self-respect, less people-pleasing, you're succeeding.

What Success Actually Looks Like

Success doesn't look like never slipping. Success looks like:

- Slipping less frequently
- Noticing when you slip
- Course correcting faster
- Not spiralling into shame when you slip
- Learning from each slip
- Getting back on track quickly
- Overall trajectory moving toward healthier patterns

That's what you're aiming for. Not perfection. Just consistent progress with occasional setbacks that you recover from.

Permission to Be Imperfect

You have permission to:

- Slip sometimes
- Make mistakes
- Backslide occasionally
- Not be perfect at this
- Still be learning years from now
- Need help
- Struggle with this

You're not a robot. You're a human trying to change deeply ingrained patterns. That's hard. Give yourself grace.

The goal is not to never slip. The goal is to slip less, learn faster, and keep going.

So when you slip, not if, when, be kind to yourself. Understand what happened. Learn from it. And get back to the work of honouring yourself.

You've got this. Even when you slip. Especially when you slip.

Keep going.

Conclusion: Honouring Yourself for Life

You made it to the end of the book. You understand the concepts now. You see how your family dynamics play out in your friendships. You recognize your tendency to lose yourself in relationships. You know why you can't set boundaries. You understand why you seek approval, avoid conflict, people-please, and sacrifice yourself constantly.

Knowledge is powerful. But it's not enough.

The real work starts now. The work of actually implementing this. Of setting boundaries and enforcing them. Of saying no without apologizing. Of choosing yourself even when it's uncomfortable. Of honouring yourself, day after day, in small moments and big decisions.

This isn't a one-time fix. This is a lifelong practice.

What You've Learned

Let's recap what we've covered:

You learned that emotional hygiene is about maintaining your emotional and relational health through consistent practices. That it's not something you do once. It's something you do daily.

You learned how family dynamics shape your adult relationships. How the roles you played as a child show up in your friendships, your romantic relationships, your workplace dynamics. How you unconsciously recreate what's familiar, even when familiar is dysfunctional.

You learned about boundaries. That they're not optional. That they're not mean or selfish. That they're the foundation of healthy relationships. That you have to set them, state them clearly, and enforce them consistently.

You learned to recognize when friendships need to end. When workplaces are toxic. When romantic relationships require you to abandon yourself. When people-pleasing is costing you your life.

You learned the difference between red flags and green flags. Between healthy love and co-dependency. Between compromise and self-abandonment.

You learned practical strategies. The 30-day reset. How to handle slips. Scripts for setting boundaries. Ways to spot your patterns and interrupt them.

But knowledge is just the beginning.

The Real Work

The real work is waking up every day and choosing yourself. It's:

- Saying no when you want to say yes to keep the peace
- Setting a boundary knowing it will disappoint someone
- Leaving a relationship that's not working, even when you're scared to be alone
- Stopping the rescue pattern with someone you love
- Letting someone be angry with you without trying to fix it

• Asking for what you need instead of hoping someone notices

• Being yourself even when it means not everyone will like you

• Choosing your wellbeing over others' comfort

Every single day, you'll face moments where you can choose yourself or abandon yourself. Where you can hold your boundary or let it slide. Where you can say the hard thing or stay quiet.

Those moments are where the real work happens. Not in reading this book. Not in understanding the concepts. In the actual daily practice of honouring yourself.

It Will Be Uncomfortable

Let's be honest: this work is uncomfortable. Changing lifelong patterns is uncomfortable. Setting boundaries with people who've never experienced your boundaries is uncomfortable. Disappointing people is uncomfortable. Being called selfish is uncomfortable. Losing relationships that can't survive your boundaries is uncomfortable.

You will feel guilty. You will feel anxious. You will feel scared. You will question yourself. You will wonder if you're being too much, too difficult, too selfish.

Feel it all. And do the work anyway.

Discomfort is not damage. Guilt doesn't mean you're wrong. Anxiety doesn't mean you should stop. Other people's disappointment doesn't mean you should cave.

The discomfort is part of the process. It's your nervous system adjusting to new patterns. It's the old programming protesting. It's normal.

Don't let discomfort stop you. Let it inform you. Let it show you where the work is needed. But don't let it dictate your choices.

You Will Lose People

Some people won't survive your boundaries. Some friendships will end. Some family relationships will become distant. Some romantic relationships will fall apart.

This is painful. This is loss. Grieve it.

But also understand: the people you lose were only in your life because you didn't have boundaries. They weren't connecting with the real you. They were connecting with your performance, your people-pleasing, your self-abandonment.

Losing people who can't handle the real you isn't actually losing anything real. It's losing illusion. It's losing dysfunction. It's making space for actual healthy relationships.

The right people, the people who are actually your people, will respect your boundaries. They'll appreciate your authenticity. They'll love you more when you're fully yourself, not less.

But you have to clear out the people who don't to make space for the people who will.

You Will Find Your People

When you stop abandoning yourself, you become available for real connection. When you stop people-pleasing, you attract people who like the real you. When you set boundaries, you filter for people who respect them.

The people who stay, the people who come into your life when you're being authentic, those are your people. They're the relationships worth investing in.

These relationships will feel different. Easier. More reciprocal. More authentic. Less exhausting. They'll energize you instead of draining you.

This is what healthy relationships feel like. This is what you deserve. This is what's waiting on the other side of your boundaries.

The Life You're Building

By practicing emotional hygiene, by honouring yourself, by setting and maintaining boundaries, you're building a different life.

A life where:

- Your needs matter as much as everyone else's
- Your time and energy are protected
- Your relationships are reciprocal and respectful
- You can be yourself without apology
- You're not constantly exhausted from managing everyone else

- You choose based on what you want, not what will keep the peace
- You're not performing for approval
- You're actually living, not just surviving

This life is possible. But you have to build it. Every boundary you set is a brick. Every time you choose yourself is another brick. Every no without apology, every hard conversation, every moment of honouring yourself. They all add up.

You're building a life that actually fits you. A life that's sustainable. A life where you're not constantly sacrificing yourself for everyone else.

Keep building.

The Permission You Need

In case you still need to hear it:

You have permission to set boundaries. You have permission to say no. You have permission to disappoint people. You have permission to choose yourself. You have permission to end relationships that don't serve you. You have permission to stop sacrificing yourself. You have permission to ask for what you need. You have permission to be imperfect at this. You have permission to take up space. You have permission to be fully yourself.

You don't need anyone else's permission. But if you're waiting for it, here it is.

You're allowed to honour yourself. You're allowed to protect yourself. You're allowed to build a life that actually works for you.

Not someday. Not when you've earned it. Not when you're perfect at it. Now. Today. You're allowed right now.

Start Today

Don't wait until you're ready. You'll never feel completely ready. Don't wait until it's easier. It won't get easier until you start practicing.

Start today. Start small if you need to. Say one no. Set one boundary. Choose yourself in one moment.

Then tomorrow, do it again. And the next day. And the next.

This is how change happens. Not in one dramatic moment. In a thousand small choices to honour yourself instead of abandoning yourself.

Start.

The Journey Ahead

This journey isn't linear. You'll have good days and bad days. Days where you hold all your boundaries and days where you slip into every old pattern. Days where you feel strong and days where you feel like you've learned nothing.

All of it is part of the process. All of it is normal. All of it is okay.

The journey is long. It's lifelong, actually. Because emotional hygiene isn't something you achieve and then you're done. It's something you practice. Every day. For the rest of your life.

But it gets easier. The boundaries get clearer. The guilt gets quieter. The people-pleasing impulse gets weaker. The choice to cherish yourself gets more automatic.

Not because you're perfect. But because you're practicing. Consistently. Imperfectly. But persistently.

You Deserve This

You deserve relationships that respect you. You deserve boundaries that are honoured. You deserve to take up space. You deserve to have needs. You deserve to say no. You deserve to be yourself. You deserve to be chosen by people who actually see you.

You deserve a life that doesn't require you to constantly abandon yourself.

Not because you've earned it by being good enough. Just because you're human. That's all the qualification you need.

You deserve this. Believe it. Act like it. Build a life that reflects it.

Final Words

Honouring yourself isn't selfish. It's essential. It's the foundation of everything else. You can't show up authentically in the world if you're constantly betraying yourself. You can't have healthy relationships if you don't have boundaries. You can't live fully if you're always making yourself smaller.

This work, the work of emotional hygiene, of setting boundaries, of choosing yourself, is some of the most important work you'll ever do. It's hard work. Uncomfortable work. Ongoing work.

But it's worth it.

You're worth it.

So go do the work. Set the boundaries. Say the nos. Choose yourself. Honor yourself. Not perfectly. Just consistently.

The life you want is on the other side of your boundaries.

Go build it

9 788169 067379

Printed at Repro India Ltd.